This book is dedicated to the evolution of humankind. No person, business, or lobby group has given me any money, favors or objects to influence the information herein. May this book help you achieve your genetic potential!
Craig B. Sommers ND, CN

"Let food be thy medicine," *Hippocrates (460-377 B.C.)*
"What people know depends on who owns the press," *Bill Moyers*

Artwork and photo credits:

Front cover design by Christina Ott, www.BareFootBuilder.com
Waterfall photo taken by Craig Sommers located on p. 2
Cloud Photo, taken by Sat Jit Kaur, located on p. 5, www.SpiralBuddy.com
Sunrise in Baja, taken by Craig Sommers, located on p. 6
Tree of Life – Summer , by Gwen Ingram, Copyright Yoga Technology, LLC, located on p. 38
Staff of Life ©, by Vivianne Nantel, www.VivianneNantel.com, 1-866-SOUL-ART, located on p. 57
Fast Food Cartoon, by Betty Seaman, located on p. 86, PO Box 500, Los Olivos, California 93441
Druids at Stonehenge, by Gwen Ingram, located on p. 94
Elephant Skies #6, Remains of the Day by Harimandir Khalsa www.Harimandir.com located on p. 111
Identical Twins cartoon, by Lou Gedo, located on p. 114, email, sexyvegan@nyc.rr.com
Woman Meditating, by Hector Jara, located on p. 120
Comic Strip throughout recipe section and cartoon of a blender located on p. 147
by Kitzia Howearth email, siempresemillas@yahoo.com

Edited by: Barry Sommers, Mark Hoffman, Justice and Deer Fields, Elaine Regan, Deborah Chambers, Linda Krall, Leonard S. Rosenbaum and Jody Foege

Published by Guru Beant Press, a division of You Can Do It Productions
Printed by Mike the Printer, email Mike@MikethePrinter.com

Printed on recycled paper, 100% post consumer content
ISBN 0-9744306-9-2
Email orders **CraigBSommers@Gmail.com**

www.RawFoodsBible.com

Table of Contents

Recipe Credits

These recipes have been designed by the top raw food chefs of North America; all are the property of the cited chef. For permission to use a recipe for commercial purposes, please contact the chef or email, RawFoodsBible@RawFoods.com for contact info.

Breakfast:

Yogurt:

Nondairy Milks and Beverages:

Pâtés:

Spreads:

Nondairy Cheeses:

Pizza Crust, Sprouted Bread, and Crackers:

Entrees:

Side Dishes:

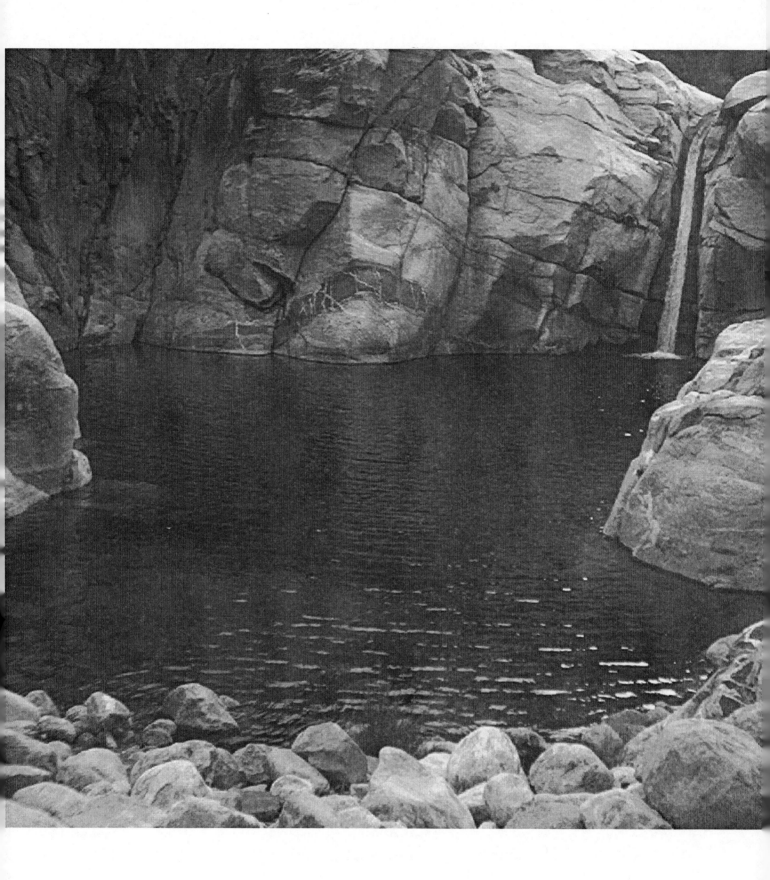

About the Author

My wake up call came in the early 1990's while visiting my mother in the hospital. That afternoon a gentleman walked into my mother's hospital room and said, "Hi, I teach people how to heal through simple diet and lifestyle changes." He handed us a business card and said to call if we wanted his help. Though I had never heard anyone say that type of thing before, I believed him because to me the idea sounded logical. My mother called him a charlatan and tossed his card in the garbage. I thought about the food that they were feeding my mother in the hospital--cholesterol-laden fatty garbage--and that she was in for clogged arteries. In that moment a seed was planted in my consciousness that was soon to blossom and consume my entire life. I set out to find the "truth," and truth I did find!

There is an old saying, "When the student is ready, the teacher will appear." My wonderful teachers began appearing in rapid succession. I researched and studied constantly. The 80 mile round-trip commute to work became a classroom for audio cassettes with teachings on alternative medicine; the VCR no longer played movies for entertainment but became a tool for learning. I began collecting books on alternative medicine and attended conferences and lectures on health-related topics whenever possible.

My mother had already survived three angioplasties, a procedure that temporarily unclogs arteries. Each time her arteries clogged again within only a few months. After the third angioplasty, she was told that she would need bypass surgery. I stepped in at that point after only a few weeks of research, got my mother on several nutritional supplements and had her cut most of the artery-clogging animal fats and processed foods out of her diet. The only animal product that she continued to consume was a moderate amount of fish. She also started eating more salads.

Within a year my mother, who was previously told that she needed blood pressure lowering drugs and had been taking cholesterol lowering medicine, an aspirin a day for its blood thinning properties, Premarin and Provera, drugs that are supposed to help hormone deficiencies, stopped her drugs. All of her lab reports showed that she no longer needed medication. Her doctor said, "I don't want to know what you're doing, but whatever you're doing keep doing it." She never had that bypass surgery.

Osteoporosis was another problem that my mother faced. In the early 1990's she had a bone density test which diagnosed osteoporosis and was told to supplement her diet with TUMS®, an over-the-counter calcium carbonate supplement. Two years later she was tested again and told that the osteoporosis had gotten worse. Her doctor tried to put her on pharmaceuticals to help strengthen her bones, but she was aware of the side effects of the drugs. Instead she chose to let me help her. The first thing I had her do was to stop taking the TUMS®, which was causing her to be constipated, and to start drinking the juices of dark green leafy vegetables every morning on an empty stomach. I sent a sample of her hair to a laboratory for a hair-mineral analysis. The lab report showed her to be deficient in magnesium but fairly high in calcium so I had her cut back on the high quality calcium supplements that she had just started and start consuming more of the high quality magnesium supplements that she had also just started, along with trace minerals such as boron. She waited eight years before receiving the next bone density test during which time I arranged a for yearly mineral analysis. The results were constant: she needed more magnesium and less calcium. She finally stopped the calcium supplements altogether. The results of her last bone density test were spectacular! She had perfect bone density, and she was now in her early seventies!

I too have benefited greatly from healthy lifestyle choices, positive thinking, and a diet of predominantly uncooked and unprocessed whole foods. Before I started on the path to healthy living, I thought that I was perfectly healthy except for dandruff, athlete's foot, small pimples on my upper arms, recurring warts on my hands, love handles, a small beer belly, pinpoint hemorrhages (small red dots) on my chest, slow-moving bowels, poor memory, a short temper, and a twenty-four hour, seven-day-a-week stuffy nose. My doctor said that none of these problems were related to my diet. I saw a registered dietitian at the medical center and was told the same thing: that none of these problems were diet related. However, when I cut out processed foods and animal products, and started eating mostly raw foods, these problems vanished! I also noticed that wounds and insect bites such as fire ants and bees, healed much more quickly. My life improved in every way possible!

I had been working in the Brooklyn College Student Center as a building mechanic for ten years. I was the shop steward for the union and had a very 'cushy' job. I could have easily stayed there until retirement, but I knew that many people were suffering and dying simply from lack of knowledge about how to achieve health, and that I could perhaps help. I went back to school to earn a degree in nutrition and opened a health food store.

Before I discovered my calling as a naturopath, I had more than 18 years of experience with plumbing and electricity, learning why pipes clog and electrical circuits fail. That experience has helped me to understand why arteries clog and how the electrical impulses in our bodies go haywire. I feel that I have been truly blessed to experience all that I have and understand all that I do. My desire now is to share that information with you so that you may help yourself and others to achieve optimum health.

During the years I spent working in my health food store on Long Island, NY, I counseled many people on their health. But the responsibilities of running a business took a toll on me and left me feeling stressed. Yoga helped, but the stress would return. I sold the store, returning to school to become a naturopath, and took a teacher-training course in Kundalini yoga. I now travel giving lectures on how to create health and provide private counseling sessions both by phone and in people's homes. Helping people stay healthy and teaching them how to regain their health is my life's work and it touches me very deeply.

I have witnessed countless people regain their health and thus improve their lives, using the information outlined in this book and I believe this information will help you too!

Introduction

The name on this book implies that it is strictly about food. It is not. There are many factors that contribute to health and disease. This book will explore three main categories of health: Nutrition, lifestyle, and the mind/body connection. Picture a three-legged stool. If one of the legs is shorter than the others the stool will be off balance or fall over. Each leg must be equal in order to achieve balance, and so it is with human health. Nutrition, lifestyle, and the mind/body connection must be balanced.

An ever-increasing number of people in the United States and worldwide refer to themselves as Raw or Living Foodists, some of which are just tired of being ill while others seek to reach their highest health potential.

In the p.s that follow, I share scientific documentation and ancient wisdom gathered from sources such as medical dictionaries, books by physicians, researchers, mystics, and even material from the Archives of the Vatican and the Old Testament.

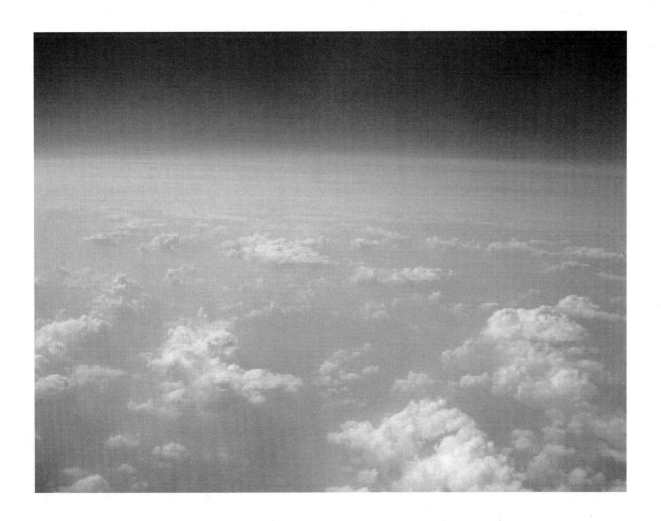

Chapter One: Nutrients, the Building Blocks of Immunity

In this chapter I am going to supply you with knowledge about the essential nutrients needed for optimum health and longevity, several of which are ignored by mainstream nutritionists.

Taber's Cyclopedic Medical Dictionary, 17th edition, defines nutrition as, "All the processes involved in the taking in and utilization of food substances by which growth, repair, and maintenance of activities in the body as a whole or in any of its parts are accomplished. Includes ingestion, digestion, absorption, and metabolism (assimilation)...". As you may gather, consuming the needed nutrient does not guarantee that the nutrient will be assimilated by the body.

Many people on this planet are aware that proper nutrition is essential for good health and that inadequate nutrition is associated with poor health and disease. Yet the corporations that control the majority of the food sold in markets are getting away with supplying very low quality products. Corporations routinely package and market foods based on their shelf life and taste rather than their nutritional value. Seed variations are selected for ease of growing, harvesting, transporting, and processing rather than nutrition. Adding chemicals to achieve a longer shelf-life is commonplace and the over refining of grains is ubiquitous. These practices contribute to inadequate nutrition which leads, in turn, to ill health.

Have you ever had someone tell you that they have a chemical imbalance? Consider the idea that they are suffering from an essential nutrient deficiency. Do you believe that a pharmaceutical can supply the missing nutrients?

Scientific research proves that many essential nutrients are destroyed in cooking; so are cooked foods still whole foods? This chapter explains why fresh, uncooked and unprocessed whole foods are the most important health guardians available to the human organism.

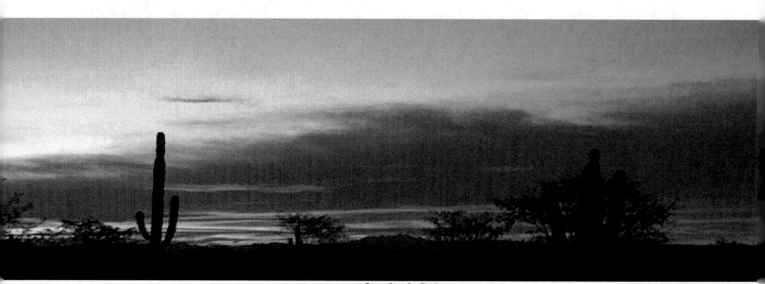

Sunrise in Baja

Enzymes

The Fourteenth Edition of *Taber's Cyclopedic Medical Dictionary* defines an enzyme as "… an organic catalyst produced by living cells but capable of acting independently. Enzymes are complex proteins that are capable of inducing chemical changes in other substances without being changed themselves. Enzymes are specific in their action. They will act only upon a certain substance or a group of closely related chemical substances and no other. Each enzyme has an optimum temperature at which it acts with greatest efficiency, and it is influenced by the reaction of the medium in which it acts, there being an optimum degree of acidity or alkalinity. Enzyme activity can be retarded or inhibited by low temperatures, high temperatures, and the presence of salts of heavy metals, dehydration, and ultraviolet radiation. Several hundred enzymes have been identified but as many as a thousand are thought to be present in mammals."

Dr. Edward Howell has been involved with enzyme research for much of his professional career, finally authoring a cutting-edge book called *Enzyme Nutrition*. In this book he states, "Life could not exist without enzymes. Enzymes convert the food we eat into chemical structures that can pass through the membranes of the cells lining the digestive tract and into the blood stream. Food must be digested so that it can ultimately pass through cell membranes. Enzymes also aid in converting the prepared food into new muscle, flesh, bone, nerves, and glands. Working with the liver, they help store excess food for future energy and building needs. They also assist the kidneys, lungs, liver, skin and colon in their important eliminative tasks. Perhaps it would be easier to write about what enzymes don't do, for they are involved in almost every aspect of life."

There are three main types of enzymes: 1) metabolic enzymes, which perform countless tasks inside our bodies, 2) digestive enzymes, which digest the foods that we eat, and 3) enzymes present in living and raw foods which initiate digestion, helping us digest our food. Metabolic and digestive enzymes are manufactured by our bodies while the enzymes present in living foods are manufactured by the plants. By consuming foods rich in live enzymes, we allow our bodies to use the energy of manufacturing digestive enzymes for other metabolic functions.

The heating of food above 118 degrees Fahrenheit destroys the naturally occurring enzymes in the food. This is of great concern to those individuals seeking optimum health and longevity because the body must work to manufacture enzymes that the cooking of the food has destroyed.

Dr. Howell writes, "All uncooked foods contain an abundance of food enzymes which correspond to the nutritional highlights of food. For example, dairy foods, oils, seeds and nuts, which are relatively high in fat content, also contain relatively higher concentrations of the enzyme lipase which aids in the digestion of their fats. Carbohydrates, such as grains, contain a higher concentration of amylase [digests carbohydrates] and lesser amounts of lipase and protease [digests protein]" (Howell p. 35).

The banana is an excellent example of how a food is capable of digesting its own ingredients. "The banana has about 20 percent starch when green. The enzyme amylase changes the banana into 20 percent sugar when the fruit is kept warm for a few days and becomes speckled. The amylase in bananas works on banana starch, but not readily on other starches, such as potato starch."

Professor Artturi Virtanen, Helsinki biochemist and Nobel Prize winner, showed that enzymes are released in the mouth from raw vegetables when they are chewed: they come into contact with the food and start digestion. These food enzymes are not denatured by stomach acid, as some researchers have speculated, but remain active throughout the digestive tract (Holford, p. 91).

So what's the big deal about getting these digestive enzymes from the diet as opposed to using the body's organs to supply the digestive enzymes? According to the research of Dr. Howell, enzyme expert, each individual has what he calls an "enzyme potential" or "enzyme bank account" and when it runs out, the organism's life ends. How does one's enzyme bank account get depleted? According to Dr. Howell, it is by "heavy withdrawals, and skimpy deposits" of enzymes.

Many researchers are now convinced that each of us is given a limited enzyme potential at birth, our genetic potential. This supply, similar to the energy supply of a new battery, has to last a lifetime. The faster you use up your enzyme supply, the shorter your life. A great deal of our enzyme energy is wasted haphazardly throughout life. The habit of cooking our food and eating it processed with chemicals, and the use of alcohol, drugs, and junk food, all draw out tremendous quantities of enzymes from our limited supply. Frequent colds and fevers and exposure to extremes of temperature also deplete the supply. A body in such a weakened, enzyme-deficient state is a prime target for cancer, obesity, heart disease, or other degenerative problems. A lifetime of such abuse ends in the tragedy of death at middle age (Howell pg. ix).

"The length of life is inversely proportional to the rate of exhaustion of the enzyme potential of an organism. The increased use of food enzymes promotes a decreased rate of exhaustion of the enzyme potential" (Howell). One of the keys to a healthy, long life is to consume dietary enzymes so that the body conserves the metabolic enzymes and uses them for other functions.

"The remarkable thing about the eventual bankruptcy of the enzyme account is that it can proceed quite painlessly, without immediate symptoms. The only warning may be a belated malfunction or a breakdown in some organ far removed from the digestive tract. But the diagnostician, unaware of the importance of enzyme nutrition, would have difficulty in connecting such a referred process to the true, underlying cause. This is how an assortment of human ailments may get started" (Howell p. 73).

Enzymes can also disarm free radicals. "Apples, mangos and grapes contain enzymes called peroxidase and catulase which help disarm free radicals" (Holford, pp. 91-92). Some mushrooms, sweet corn and raw honey also contain these enzymes along with amylase. However, when these foods are cooked, the beneficial enzymes are destroyed.

Some foods contain enzyme inhibitors. For example, lentils, beans and chickpeas contain trypsin-inhibitors that prevent protein from being completely digested. However, this anti-enzyme factor can be destroyed either by sprouting or cooking. The same is true for grains rich in phytates that can bind beneficial minerals. If these enzyme blockers are not inactivated, they can create an enzyme drain on the body and cause intestinal gas. Nuts with brown skins, such as almonds, contain enzyme inhibitors. Soaking the nuts from 8 to 12 hours depending on the type of nut deactivates these inhibitors.

"Previously, food was considered to have no effects except for the production of heat and energy from fats and carbohydrates and the repair of tissue by proteins. Now it is known that food can change organs and tissues, including glands, for better or worse. The fact that food can change the size and weight of these important glands, such as the pituitary, testicles, ovaries, pancreas, adrenal, and thyroid, has been demonstrated over and over again by careful experiments during past years. Professor Jackson and co-workers at the University of Minnesota fed white rats a diet containing 80 percent sugar (enzyme free) and reported marked differences in the size and weight of all principal organs and glands" (Howell p. 104).

"Heat-treated, enzyme-free refined items of food caused the most drastic deviations in pituitary gland size and appearance. **When animals were fed diets greatly restricted in enzymes, the damage in the pituitary was identical or similar to that found in human beings subsisting on conventional food** with greatly lowered food enzyme intake" (Howell p. 106). The *Taber's Cyclopedic Medical Dictionary*, 17th edition (p. 1516) says the following about the function of the pituitary gland: "The pituitary is an endocrine gland secreting a number of hormones that regulate many bodily processes, including growth, reproduction, and various metabolic activities. It is often referred to as the master gland of the body...". It has been proven that a predominantly cooked-food diet can make one's "master gland" a gland that regulates so many bodily functions, shrink! Do you think that this could be a contributing factor in the cause of some of the diseases of modern society? Many researchers do.

Dr. Howell explains how a predominately cooked-food diet causes an enlargement of the pancreas. "The pancreas must send messages to all parts of the body looking for enzymes it can reprocess into digestive enzymes. It may even invade the warehouse of the precursors. In a pinch it will beg, borrow or steal them. When it finds them it has work to do. Changing metabolic enzymes into digestive enzymes means extra work for the pancreas. It must get bigger, just as muscle grows from more exercise... Either way, your brain, heart, arteries, all organs and tissues suffer from an enzyme labor shortage" (Howell p. 81). The pancreas also must secrete insulin to deal with the massive amounts of processed sugar that the average person consumes nowadays. This combination of enzyme-free food and a large amount of processed sugar leads to the overburdening of the pancreas which can then lead to enlargement and dangerous disease of this organ.

Dr. Howell has assessed more than fifty reports submitted in scientific periodical literature on nutrition and brain weight over a number of years. **He found that animals fed a diet "armed to the hilt with various vitamins and**

9

minerals," but completely free of food enzymes had consistently lower brain weights than animals fed a diet consisting of a mixture of cooked and uncooked foods (Howell, p. 76).

I hardly ever indulge in cooked foods, but when I do, I consume a dietary supplement of **plant-based enzymes** in veggie capsules. These pills help me digest the enzyme-free food so that my body does not have to generate as many digestive enzymes, therefore lessening the strain on my digestive system. If you decide to supplement your diet with digestive enzymes, beware of animal-based enzymes. They may come from the pancreas of a pig or other animal. These enzymes only work in a particular pH, unlike plant enzymes which work under a broad range of acidity or alkalinity, as do our stomachs. Another factor is that animals carry disease, and enzymes that come from an animal cannot be sterilized because the heat would destroy the enzymes, so they could possibly cause us more harm than good. For these two reasons I suggest the use of plant-based enzymes.

Vitamins

Vitamins are organic substances which the body requires in small amounts to carry out thousands of building-up and breaking-down functions. Many scientific studies have shown that a high dietary intake of vitamins is associated with health and a low dietary intake of vitamins is associated with disease.

Unfortunately, the vitamins in our foods are often rendered inactive before we get a chance to consume them. The *Taber's Cyclopedia Medical Dictionary*, Edition 17 (p. 1562) has this to say about vitamin loss: "...loss of vitamin content [occurs] in food products because of vitamin instability, especially in oxidation and during heating. Methods of preserving foods add to the loss of vitamins. Pickling, salting, curing or fermenting processes usually cause complete loss of Vitamin C. Commercial canning destroys from fifty to eighty-five percent of Vitamin C contained in peas, lima beans, spinach and asparagus. Pasteurization, unless special precautions are observed, causes a loss of from thirty to sixty percent of Vitamin C. Freshly prepared applesauce retains only from twenty to thirty percent of the Vitamin C value of the apple. Vitamin B1 is lost through milling because the wheat embryo, rich in Vitamin B1, is removed from wheat flour in milling. Some vitamins are unstable, being readily destroyed by oxidation, heat, especially in an alkaline medium or strong acids, light and aging."

The Vitamin Chart in this prestigious medical dictionary states the following (edition 14, p. 1725, except where otherwise indicated).

- **Vitamin A**, "**destroyed by high temperatures** when oxygen is present."
- **Vitamin B1**, "**destroyed by exposure to heat,** alkali or sulphites."
- **Vitamin B2**, "unstable in light, especially in the presence of alkali."
- **Vitamin B6**, "**rapidly inactivated in the presence of heat,** sunlight, or air."
- **Vitamin B12**, "unstable in hot alkaline or acid solutions" (edition 19, p. 2399).

- **Folic Acid**, "**destroyed by heat** at low pH, loss in food stored at room temperature" (edition 19, p. 2399).
- **Vitamin C**, "easily destroyed by oxidation; heat hastens the process. **Lost in cooking**, particularly if water in which food is cooked is discarded. Also loss is greater if cooked in iron or copper utensils."
- **Vitamin E**, "**destroyed by heat**" (edition 19, p 2399).

I am of the belief that we should meet our daily vitamin needs by the consumption of living and whole foods. However, there is one vitamin that I must recommend that everyone supplement, B12. Although B12 deficiencies occur more often in vegetarians and vegans, they also occur in non-vegetarians. Vitamin B12 deficiencies are associated with elevated homocysteine (along with B6 and folic acid). Research has shown that elevated homocysteine increases the potential for deterioration of the arteries and nerves and several other unfavorable conditions. The nerve system degeneration that can occur from B12 deficiency can sometimes be irreversible. Symptoms include numbness and tingling in the hands and feet, poor memory, behavioral changes such as paranoia and nervousness, and impotence.

Gabriel Cousens, M.D. explains that the minimal need for B12 is about 6 micrograms (mcg) per day and that we lose about 3 mcg per day. Furthermore, he adds that 80 percent of children, adult vegans and live-food practitioners become B12 deficient after six to ten years without B12 supplementation (Cousens pg. 285).

I use a form of B12 called methylcobalamin in a sublingual lozenge. My typical dose is 1000 mcg once per week.

What about food sources for B12? Sea vegetables do contain some human active B12. Unfortunately they also contain an analog form of B12 that can block receptor sites for human active B12. For this reason I do not suggest that anyone rely on sea vegetables for B12. Dr. Cousens states in his book *Conscious Eating* that Vitamin B12 is heat-sensitive but not entirely destroyed by cooking. Research has shown that between 23.7% and 96.4% of B12 is destroyed by boiling or baking, depending on the type of food and cooking duration. Nutritional yeast (Red Star brand) seems to be a source for B12 but supplements are undoubtedly the best way to ensure adequate consumption.

Vitamin C is a very interesting vitamin. Practically all animals make it in their bodies so they don't have to eat it. The exceptions are fruit-eating bats, guinea pigs, the red-vented bulbous bird and primates including humans. Linus Pauling, a famous Vitamin C researcher, postulated that humans once made it. However, from eating a fruit-rich diet, we lost the ability to produce it. Diets high in food-derived Vitamin C have been proven to reduce the risk of heart disease and cancer which are currently the top causes of death in the United States.

Today it is widely known that if we don't get Vitamin C through our diets, we develop scurvy. In 1747, James Lind, a British physician discovered that fresh fruit was the cure for scurvy. Yet it wasn't until the early 1800's that the government recognized this and started putting citrus fruits on their ships. The death of sailors by scurvy continued for many years while health experts failed to convince the ruling powers to include citrus in sailors' diets. (In 1907 Vitamin C was officially recognized as the cure and prevention of scurvy.) If our society could learn from the mistakes of our predecessors and recognize the vast body of scientific evidence that points to a whole foods diet as the prevention of most modern diseases, it would save countless people from suffering and premature death.

Vitamin D is known as the "sunshine" vitamin. In other words, when our bodies are exposed to sunlight (usually twenty minutes is sufficient), we are supplied with our daily need for Vitamin D. A baby can get all the Vitamin D it needs with only its cheeks exposed to the sun for about twenty minutes daily.

The Vitamin E Fact Book by the Vitamin E Research and Information Service (1989) states that almonds are a rich source of Vitamin E in their raw state but they lose eighty percent of the vitamin in roasting.

Large numbers of illnesses can be caused by vitamin deficiencies. Just to name a few: lack of Vitamin A can cause the eyes to weaken; lack of Vitamin B3 can cause pellagra; lack of Vitamin C can cause scurvy; and lack of Vitamin D can cause rickets. The government has set dietary recommendations (RDA's) for these vitamins to prevent deficiency diseases, but most researchers believe that RDA recommendations are less than optimal. Every individual has a different need for vitamins that changes constantly according to lifestyle factors. Water-soluble vitamins, if over-ingested, will usually leave the body through the urine and not cause any problems. Fat-soluble vitamins such as A, D, E and K, are stored in the liver and fatty tissues until the body needs them. For this reason the body can survive weeks of consuming foods that lack them without any deficiency signs. However, the capacity for storage sets the stage for toxic build-up should an excess be ingested.

Storage of vitamins A, D and K can easily reach toxic levels if over consumed. For example, a man driving an Alaskan dog sled got lost, and in an attempt to save himself from death, the stranded man ate the liver of one of the dogs and then died of Vitamin A toxicity. If, however, a human ate an excess of plant foods, toxic levels of vitamin A would never be reached because plants contain carotinoids that are changed into vitamin A only as the body needs them.

Synergistic and opposing relationships exist between some vitamins. For example, Vitamins A, D and E are mutually antagonistic to each other, and it is well known that hyper-vitaminosis A can be treated by Vitamin D supplementation. In addition, an excess of Vitamin D in the body can be successfully treated with Vitamin A supplementation. An excess of the mineral calcium in the body can cause a Vitamin A deficiency, and a deficiency of the mineral zinc can prevent the body from accessing Vitamin A stored in the liver. Vitamin D can become deficient if excess magnesium is present. Thus indiscriminate supplementation or eating an excess of fortified foods can cause imbalance. Foods in their natural state as the Creator has designed them (i.e. excluding excessively hybridized and genetically modified foods), have the vitamins and minerals in highly usable ratios. Normal consumption of a good variety of foods does not cause imbalance. However, if we eat refined and processed foods that have been enriched with synthetic vitamins and laboratory-manipulated minerals and then consume synthetic supplemental vitamins in high doses, body chemistry can become imbalanced. If you use supplemental vitamins, be sure to use quality products from a health food store and never from discount stores, pharmacies or supermarkets. Sometimes these supplements contain artificial chemicals that can cause ill health.

According to research done by Dr. David L. Watts, some vitamins have been classified as having either a stimulating or sedating effect at the cellular level. For most people, vitamins A, C, E, B1, B3, B6 and B10 are stimulators while vitamins D and B2 are sedatives. I have often wondered if the high dose of vitamin D absorbed from the sun is the reason why most people feel so sedated after a day at the beach.

Minerals

Seventeen of the thirty elements known to be essential to life are metals. These metals act as signal transducers for activation of different DNA expressions (Cousens pg. 311).

Mineral deficiencies cause disease in humans. For example, goiter, an enlargement of the thyroid gland (in the throat), can be caused by a deficiency of the mineral iodine. When Iodine is added to the diet, the goiter goes away.

Mineral toxicity is widely recognized. The problems in children who eat peeling lead-based paints and suffer lead toxicity is an example. Many historians believe lead poisoning contributed to the fall of the Roman Empire.

Eleonore Blaurock-Busch, PhD states in her book, *Mineral and Trace Element Analysis*, **"Selenium compounds are unstable and loss of the mineral occurs during cooking."** Selenium is a very important mineral that our bodies use in many ways. The following is a list of symptoms of selenium deficiency (from the same book): cataracts, calcium deposits in muscle tissue, elevated cholesterol levels, increased susceptibility to cancer, mercury and cadmium poisoning, growth impairment, poor resistance to infection, reduced tissue levels of coenzyme Q10, and necrotic changes in the liver. I eat Brazil nuts for selenium and raw wheat germ can be a good source if the wheat is grown in selenium-rich soil.

Zinc is another mineral that some sources say becomes unstable in and is destroyed by high temperature cooking. Zinc is essential for the proper functioning of more than 300 enzymes (Cousins pg. 311).

Many countries around the world have restricted the use of mercury amalgam dental fillings, also called silver fillings. Japan, Sweden, Denmark, Norway and Canada have stopped using amalgam filling. What do these countries have in common? Health care paid for by the government. There has been extensive research done at the University of Calgary on the safety of amalgam fillings. Much of this research has been documented on a video called *Smoking Teeth*. Here are three significant findings from that body of research. They put amalgam dental fillings into the teeth of small animals and then autopsied these animals several months later. They found that the mercury vapor leaching from the fillings had migrated into many of the animal's organs. In another study they had a molar from a person that had an amalgam filling in that tooth for 25 years. The tooth had been removed from the mouth and warmed in water to body temperature. Then they held the tooth in front of a phosphorescent screen. That type of screen allows us to see mercury vapor that is otherwise invisible to the human eye. When they rubbed the amalgam filling with a pencil eraser, to simulate chewing, the mercury vapor was quite visible. It looked as if someone had blown out a candle and one was viewing the candle smoke. The last piece of research from the University of Calgary showed what happens when very small amounts of mercury come in contact with our brain. They had brain cells in a Petri dish and added a very small amount of mercury. The neurite membrane that extended out from the brain cells underwent rapid degeneration. Some researchers now believe that the forgetfulness and other unfavorable changes in the brains of some elderly people may be from the mercury vapor that is constantly leaching from the fillings and the body's inability to constantly deal with the toxic burden.

According to Florida's Environmental Regulation Agency, the amount of mercury in one dental filling, if put into a ten-acre lake, would pollute that lake so dangerously that the lake would have to be closed to swimming, boating and fishing. The question here is why mercury is routinely used in dental fillings for both children and adults. They call it a mercury-amalgam filling and claim that it is safe. But mercury levels in the bloodstream rise over time as the filling leaches tiny amounts of this toxic mineral. I have had my mercury levels checked before and after replacing my mercury-amalgam fillings, and found that the mercury level in my body dropped to a safe level after removing the fillings whereas before the mercury level was dangerously high. My dental records and mineral test results are evidence of this. For this reason I suggest using other types of dental fillings if you have a cavity in a tooth. I also suggest the safe removal of amalgam fillings from the human body. Safely removing a mercury-amalgam filling means that the Dentist uses a 'dental dam' in your mouth to catch the mercury particles and equips you with a respirator to prevent you from inhaling the mercury fumes released from drilling into the fillings.

Fluoride is another controversial element that is covered in the *Personal Care Products* section of this book.

Many disease conditions caused by mineral imbalances are not commonly known. Providing sufficient minerals for a person is complicated by the fact that every person has a different need for each mineral at any given stage in his or her life. It has been said that "one man's medicine is another man's poison". Minerals have been called a double-edged sword because too much of a mineral can be just as harmful as not enough.

Since 1996, I have been working with Trace Elements Inc., a laboratory that determines mineral imbalances in humans and animals. This laboratory uses sophisticated equipment that dissolves human hair into a solution and then accurately measures the toxic and nutrient minerals that are present in the hair. Hair holds an excellent history of the minerals that have traveled through the bloodstream over the time that it took for a length of hair to grow. Through this process, I have helped many people regain their health by recommending ways for them to balance mineral ratios (body chemistry) through their diet. For more information go to www.rawfoodsbible.com and click the link labeled Hair Mineral Analysis.

The synergistic and opposing relationships between various minerals, and between vitamins and minerals, are complex. Calcium and phosphorus work synergistically in bone formation if the two minerals are in proper balance. However, when either one is consumed in excess of the other, a problem with bone formation can occur. Soda and carbonated water contain phosphoric acid to keep the bubbles in solution. Consumption of these man-made fluids can overload the body with phosphorus and lead to bone-density problems. Animal products are high in phosphorous and can cause this problem as well.

Magnesium can become deficient if an excess of vitamin D exists in the body. According to many experts as well as my own clinical experience, magnesium deficiencies are quite common. Magnesium is crucial for many very important processes in the body, including building bone and increasing bone density. I find that when I spend more time in the sun, my need for magnesium increases. (As explained in the Vitamin section, Vitamin D comes from the sun.) An excess of Vitamin D absorbed from spending time in the sun is antagonistic to the magnesium in your body.

Because of the adversarial relationship between Vitamin D and magnesium, I believe that the consumption of Vitamin D found in enriched cow's milk might lead to magnesium deficiency. Calcium and magnesium also have a synergistic and opposing relationship. Because cow's milk is very high in calcium and low in magnesium, consuming dairy products can lead to a magnesium deficiency. This fact contradicts the widely espoused notion that consuming large amounts of calcium through dairy products is the best way to fight osteoporosis. Whenever you consume large amounts of calcium without including balancing amounts of magnesium, along with other minerals and Vitamin D, as often happens when you consume large amounts of dairy products, you actually lose bone density. The Harvard Nurses Health Study (see www.PCRM.org), a twelve-year health study, consisting of 78,000 female nurses, showed that those who drank one glass of cow's milk per day ran a 1½ times greater risk of hip fracture than those who drank 1 glass or less per week.

Countries with the highest dairy intakes have the highest osteoporosis rates while countries with the lowest dairy intake have the lowest osteoporosis rates. For example, Finland, Sweden, England and the USA have the highest rates of dairy consumption and also have the highest rates of osteoporosis. Black South Africans only consume about 196 mg of calcium per day; African Americans consume much higher amounts but have a nine times greater rate of hip fracture. Calcium intake of people in rural China is 1/2 that of the USA, but the bone fracture rate of the people in rural China is 1/5 that of the USA. Sixty-five percent of all adults world-wide do not drink cow's milk, and they have strong bones! Phosphates found in milk, cheeses and eggs reduce iron absorption. So why do we see advertisements for cow's milk everywhere in the United States? Perhaps the $190 million dollars spent annually by the dairy industry on the *milk mustache* advertisements has something to do with it. But don't take my word for it. Do some research and see for yourself!

According to the research of Dr. David L. Watts, some minerals have either stimulating or sedative properties. Stimulating minerals include phosphorous, sodium, potassium, iron, selenium, manganese, chromium, and molybdenum. The following minerals have a sedative effect on most people: calcium, magnesium, zinc, copper, boron, cobalt, barium, silicon, and vanadium.

For example, many of my clients who suffer from tight and painful muscles and/or constipation are deficient in magnesium. When magnesium is added to their diet, the tight muscles or constipation often vanish! Magnesium relaxes the muscles at the cellular level.

The best sources for minerals that I am aware of are **organic** fruits and vegetables, especially sea vegetables (see "Ocean-Grown Foods" in chapter 3), with the dark green leafy veggies being the most important. The fastest way to get minerals into your body is to juice the fruits and vegetables and drink the nutrient-rich juice, or to consume powdered cereal grasses such as wheat grass, barley grass, kamut and alfalfa mixed with liquid. These dried cereal grasses are known as 'super foods'. When I consume them, they make me feel...Super!

Phytonutrients

Phytonutrients are nutrients from plant sources. This topic could fill many large books, but I will keep it brief. We should not assume that all the nutritive factors of foods are well known or understood. New nutrients are being discovered all the time. So, when we process or cook the foods that come in perfect form from nature, what else is being destroyed in addition to what is known?

Dr. L. Newman, author of *Make Your Juicer Your Drug Store*, writes, "One of the major discoveries in nutritional research was that nature never gives us isolated minerals and vitamins. She always gives them to us in combinations. Man probably does not comprehend one millionth of what still remains unknown in the field. We do know, however, that when we do fair [obtain], these vital elements from the master chemist, we are obtaining, besides the known vitamins, vitamins that have not yet been discovered."

Following are the words on the first p. of *Prescription for Nutritional Healing*, Third Edition, which claims to be America's #1 Guide to Natural Health, and which is probably the most popular and widely used book of its kind in the United States. "One problem most of us have is that we do not get the nutrients we need from our diet because most of the foods we consume are cooked and/or processed. Cooking at high temperatures and processing destroys vital nutrients the body needs to function properly. The organic raw foods that supply these elements are largely missing from today's diet." (Balch and Balch pg. 2)

Many important nutrients exist in plant foods, many of which we have not yet identified, and these nutrients can be destroyed in processing and cooking are two of the many reasons that I believe optimum health requires the consumption of a wide variety of unprocessed and uncooked plant foods.

Protein

According to the Max Planck Institute for Nutritional Research in Germany, protein, when cooked, is only 50 percent bioavailable. In other words, about half the amino acids, the building blocks of protein, are unusable by the body because they are destroyed by cooking.

The World Health Organization recommends that 5 percent of one's total daily calories come from protein. This level is easily reached on a plant-based diet. For example, 9 percent of calories in an orange are derived from protein, from zucchini 17 percent, strawberries 8, broccoli 42, cauliflower 31 and corn 13. The fact is that the commonly consumed plant foods contain 6 to 45 percent of their calories as protein. This research comes from John McDougall, M.D. He says, "Protein is so abundant in plant foods that it is impossible for any dietician or scientist to design a diet that is composed of unprocessed plant foods (starches and vegetables) and, at the same time, be deficient in protein. We would not have survived as a species if this were not true."

In the book, *Disease-Proof Your Child*, Joel Fuhrman, M.D. states, "Protein is ubiquitous; it is contained in all foods, not only animal products. Protein deficiency in not a concern for anyone in the developed world. It is almost impossible to consume too little protein, no matter what you eat... ".

All proteins are formed by amino acids joined together in specific sequences. Eight are said to be essential to adults, and ten essential to infants. The belief that one must eat all essential amino acids at every meal (also called the complete protein theory) in order to maintain health is a myth. The Wendt Doctrine, describing thirty years of research, debunks the complete protein myth. It proves that we have the ability to store these proteins in our cells and to convert them into amino acids that move freely throughout the body to areas that might be deficient. Therefore, combining beans and rice to supply complex protein is unnecessary. The Wendt Doctrine also shows the damaging effects of excess concentrated protein which clogs the system, depleting the cells of oxygen and nutrition and creates an acidic environment, a condition that eventually leads to degenerative diseases.

The Physicians Committee for Responsible Medicine (PCRM) states that, "...the average American takes in twice the amount of protein he or she needs. Excess protein has been linked with osteoporosis, kidney disease, calcium stones in the urinary tract and some cancers."

In the February 2004 issue of *Readers Digest*, in an article entitled *Kicking Kidney Stones*, the author states: "The simplest fix is to avoid high-protein diets." Then the author explains how kidney stones are formed: "Protein from meat and other animal products is broken down into acids. It's your kidney's job to balance acids with bases for elimination from the body. The handiest base is the calcium in your bones. Protein is broken down and stored in the bone, where it binds with calcium. Then the kidneys filter these particles from your blood. And the more meat you eat, the more calcium you'll have in your kidneys. Over time, these particles bind together, forming stones."

According to Leslie and Susannah Kenton, in their book, *Raw Energy*, grilling a steak at 239 degrees Fahrenheit completely destroys the amino acids lysine and cystine. Many researchers believe that the reason more people don't get extremely ill from high-protein diets is due to the fact that about 50 percent of the protein is destroyed by cooking.

Because a diet rich in a variety of plant foods can provide all the protein one needs, I see no need to worry about getting enough protein unless poor digestion and absorption is an issue. In that case, thorough chewing, supplemental digestive enzymes and intestinal cleansing can help.

Fiber

Fiber is essential for human health and a shortage of it in the diet can promote many disorders of the digestive tract. The fiber in food helps slow down digestion, keeping blood sugar stable and hunger at bay. Colon and rectal cancer are the second leading cause of death in the United States. Fiber helps to prevent colorectal cancer, constipation, diverticulosis and most other illnesses of the lower bowel. Fiber also slows the absorption of sugar and is, therefore, beneficial to diabetics and hypoglycemics. Even people who are eating diets high in fiber-rich cooked vegetables might not be getting the fiber they need to prevent these diseases because the fiber is partially destroyed by cooking.

All animal products (i.e. beef, chicken, lamb, pig, fish and shellfish, turkey, goat, etc.) completely lack fiber. All dairy products (i.e. milk, cheese, yogurt, butter, etc.) are also fiberless. Nor do eggs contain fiber. On the other hand all fruits, vegetables, beans, nuts, seeds and grains contain ample amounts of fiber in their whole and unprocessed state.

Egg whites and dairy products, as well as wheat protein (gluten) cause constipation. When wheat grain is processed into flour, the fiber is taken out, along with most of the nutrition. Many people become addicted to this fast source of carbohydrates which is lacking in nutrients.

Modern statistics show that in Africa, the average diet has approximately seven times more fiber than the American diet; colon/rectal problems are rare there, while they are commonplace in the United States.

Even the Quaker Oats Company is aware of the medical benefits of fiber and is using them to market their product to a population plagued by the effects of a diet high in fiberless animal food and low in unprocessed sources of fiber. I found the following written on a box of Quaker Oats: "Three grams of soluble fiber from oatmeal daily in a diet low in saturated fat and cholesterol may reduce the risk of heart disease. This cereal has two grams per serving." The soluble fiber in oats binds with cholesterol-based acids and prevents these acids from being absorbed into the bloodstream.

Taber's Cyclopedic Medical Dictionary (edition 14) gives a good definition of dietary fiber and outlines many of its functions.

"Components of food that are resistant to chemical digestion include portions of food that are made up of cellulose, hemi-cellulose, lignin and pectin. These substances add bulk to the diet by absorbing large amounts of water and are used in diets to produce large bulky bowel movements. Foods rich in fiber include whole grains, bran flakes, fruits, leafy vegetables, root vegetables and their skins, and prunes, which also contain a laxative substance, diphenylisatin.

Diets high in fiber may help to prevent diverticula of the intestinal tract, may help to lower blood cholesterol and possibly prevent cancer of the intestinal tract (emphasis added). Some diabetic individuals on low insulin doses have been able to further lower their insulin requirements by following a diet high in fiber and carbohydrates and low in sucrose."

While diverticula are common in people on the standard American diet, they are rare in peoples of the world who eat high fiber diets. My parents were told by their allopathic doctor that everyone gets diverticula of the intestinal tract when they get old and that there is no way to prevent it. Yet the medical dictionary states that a high fiber diet "may help to prevent diverticula of the intestinal tract" and studies have shown that diverticula are rare in places where humans consume a high fiber diet. Dr. Neil Painter, a London surgeon, was the researcher who finally proved that diverticula are caused by a fiber-deficient diet, but for 50 years before his 1972 landmark study, diverticula was treated with a low fiber diet.

If you choose to use a fiber supplement rather then getting your fiber from raw fruits and vegetables as I recommend, you should know that psyllium fiber supplements absorb about forty times their weight in water. If there is not a sufficient amount of water in the intestines to hydrate the fiber, it will dry out the intestines and cause constipation. Some supermarket brands of fiber contain artificial colors that are known to cause cancer.

I recommend using ground flax seeds for a fiber supplement. In addition to being highly nutritious, they are about 50 percent nonsoluble fiber and 50 percent soluble so they absorb less water than psyllium fiber. These seeds also contain flax oil which lubricates the intestines. Use a coffee bean grinder to pulverize them because the human digestive tract cannot break them down unless they are chewed very thoroughly. After the flax seeds are ground they must be kept either refrigerated or frozen or they will become rancid. Gandhi once commented that the people in the villages he visited (in India) that consumed flax seeds were noticeably healthier than the people in the villages that did not consume flax seeds.

Essential Fats

Essential fats and fatty acids are extremely important for health and vitality. Essential fat deficiencies are correlated with degenerative diseases including cardiovascular disease, cancer, diabetes, multiple sclerosis, skin afflictions, dry skin, premenstrual syndrome, behavioral problems, poor wound healing, arthritis, glandular atrophy, weakened immune functions and sterility (especially in males) (Udo Erasmus Ph.D., *Fats that Heal, Fats that Kill*).

Taber's Cyclopedic Medical Dictionary (17th edition) says the following about essential fatty acids: "The unsaturated fatty acids cannot be synthesized in the body and have been considered to be essential to maintain health."

Two absolutely essential fatty acids are alpha linolenic acid (omega 3) and linoleic acid (omega 6). These essential fatty acids must be provided in the diet.

Mary G. Enig, Ph.D., speaks of conditionally essential fats in her book, *Know Your Fats*. "The conditionally essential fatty acids include gamma-linolenic acid (GLA), arachidonic acid (AA), eicosapentaenoic acid (EPA), and docosahexaenoic acid (DHA). All four of these fatty acids can be made by cells in the body, but there are a number of interfering food substances, illnesses or genetic inadequacies that make these fatty acids become dietary essential for some." Our bodies convert Omega 3 into EPA, and DHA and Omega 6 into GLA and AA. The enzyme that makes it possible to convert them is called Delta 6 Desaturase. There are also nutrients needed in the conversion process. These include: zinc, magnesium, Vitamins B3, B6, and Vitamin C. There are some food substances that can interfere and slow the conversion process if consumed in excess. These food substances are: trans-fatty acids, saturated fats, cholesterol and carbohydrates.

"Every living cell in the body needs essential fatty acids. They are essential for rebuilding and producing new cells. Essential fatty acids are also used by the body for the production of prostaglandins, hormone-like substances that act as chemical messengers and regulators of various body processes" (Balch and Balch pg. 68).

The *Medline Medical Database* (1999) a review of 1757 peer-reviewed articles, lists afflictions associated with a deficiency of omega 3 fatty acids (while an omega 3 deficiency may not be the cause of the following afflictions, it has been shown to be a contributing factor). These include acne, AIDS, allergies, Alzheimer's, angina, atherosclerosis, arthritis, autoimmunity, behavioral disorders, breast cancer, breast cysts, breast pain, cancer, dementia, diabetes, eczema, heart disease, high blood pressure, hyperactivity, infection, immune deficiencies, inflammatory conditions, intestinal disorders, kidney disease, learning disorders, leukemia, lupus, malnutrition, menopause, mental illness, metastasis, multiple sclerosis, neurological disease, obesity, post viral fatigue, psoriasis, Reyes syndrome, schizophrenia, stroke, and vision disorders.

Essential fatty acids (EFAs) have desirable effects on many disorders. They improve the skin and hair, reduce blood pressure, aid in the prevention of arthritis, lower cholesterol and triglyceride levels, and reduce the risk of blood clot formation. They are beneficial for candidiasis, cardiovascular disease, eczema and psoriasis and are found in high concentrations in the brain. EFAs aid in the transmission of nerve impulses and are needed for the normal development and functioning of the brain. A deficiency of EFAs can lead to an impaired ability to learn and recall information.

Experts agree: "Heat destroys essential fatty acids. Worse, it results in the creation of dangerous free radicals" (Balch and Balch pg. 68). Udo Erasmus says, "heat destroys EFAs and turns them into poisonous breakdown products that interfere with EFA functions and create free radicals." The bottom line is: eat only living foods and you will never have to worry about consuming these poisonous breakdown products or this type of free radical that can be so damaging to the body.

One of the most knowledgeable people on the subject of EFAs, Udo Erasmus Ph.D., states, "… **all whole, fresh, unprocessed foods contain some EFA**".

"Alpha-linolenic acid (omega 3) is found in high amounts in flax, flax seed oil (approximately 60 percent) and walnut oil (10 percent). Other oils that have high levels of alpha-linolenic acid are perilla oil and hemp oil" (*Know Your Fats* by Mary G. Eniglish, Ph.D., p. 238). With the exception of fish, animal products are deficient in omega-3 fats.

"Linoleic acid (Omega 6) is found in large amounts in **unrefined** sunflower seed oil (68 percent)" (Mary G. Enig, Ph.D., *Know Your Fats*, pg. 256). I often add a tablespoon of ground flax seeds or chia seeds to a smoothie to insure my omega 3 intake. For the omega 6, I eat usually eat raw sunflower seeds. Hemp seeds are a great source of both omega 3 and omega 6 EFAs and I often consume them as well. Hemp seeds can be bought in a health food store. Be sure to refrigerate after opening.

"The daily requirement for essential fatty acids is satisfied by an amount equivalent to 10 to 20 percent of total caloric intake" (*Prescription for Nutritional Healing* by Phyllis A. Balch, CNC, and James F. Balch, M.D., pg. 69). This requirement translates into approximately two tablespoons of flax seed oil per day.

Traveling in New Zealand in 2002, I came across a sticker on an avocado that caught my attention: "*NZ AVOCADOS NATIONAL HEART FOUNDATION APPROVED.*" Just a few years prior I had suggested that my mother include small amounts of avocado in her diet. She told me that her cardiologist had told her to avoid avocados but had not told her anything about essential fats. So, who is correct: The New Zealand Heart Foundation or my mom's American cardiologist? Research on the benefits of avocados is located in the Food as Medicine section.

Chapter Two: Selected Research

Animal Studies

There are many animal studies that I will talk about, but first I would like to tell you a story about an experience I had with an animal on a raw food diet.

In November of 2003, I moved in with a friend who had had a companion rabbit for a little over two years. This rabbit, which she called "Dust Bunny," spent most of his time under the bed. He would come out to use the litter box and eat, and then return to lying under the bed. When I looked under the bed, he reminded me of how I felt after a large meal of cooked food. Dust Bunny lived on a diet consisting of about 50 percent dry pellets (these were pork free, as most rabbit pellets have pork in them) and 50 percent conventional produce.

After a month, I asked Dust Bunny's caretaker if I could try an experiment. I would feed the rabbit 100 percent raw foods. These consisted of mostly weeds and some leafy greens from a nearby organic garden, all of which I picked with my own hands, so I knew that they were fresh. He started to eat ravenously at first, sometimes eating a whole grocery bag full of greens in one day. He also became much more active, and after a week or so, would run up to me as I entered the room and put his head on my foot. The ravenous eating binge slowed after a few weeks and stopped after a month, when he began to eat a more normal amount for his size (four pounds).

His behavior became increasingly more outgoing. It became so that I had to look down with every step because he would run under my feet, and he hopped around the room begging for affection. After about five weeks, he started to venture out of the bedroom for the first time in his life (though the door had always been open)! His caretaker was very pleased, and said, "This is what I thought having a house rabbit was going to be like!" First he began walking down the hallway. A few days later he was trotting, and soon after that he was running down the hallway and finally running and leaping through the air! Finally, Dust Bunny, whom I gave the name Rascal, began frequenting the living room. Some mornings he would trot circles around me as I did my morning yoga set.

One evening there were many guests in the apartment. Rascal entered the living room and came to see what was going on. One of the guests asked, with full sincerity, "Did you get a new rabbit?" "No," my friend replied, "we just put him on a new diet". The guest said, "I took care of that rabbit once for a week and this is the first time I've actually seen him." Another guest commented, "I've slept over here lots of times and never saw the rabbit come out from under the bed before." I smiled and knew that the raw wild food diet had worked.

Many thousands of laboratory animals have been experimented on and they all prove the same point. Raw foods provide a health-promoting diet and an all-cooked-food diet promotes disease.

In India, Sir Robert McCarrison fed monkeys a cooked version of their usual diet. All the monkeys developed colitis. Post mortem examinations revealed gastric and intestinal ulcers.

In Switzerland, O. Stiner fed guinea pigs a cooked version of their usual diet. These animals quickly succumbed to anemia, scurvy, goiter, dental cavities, and degeneration of the salivary glands. When 10 CCs of pasteurized milk was added to their daily diet, they developed arthritis as well. Calves that are fed pasteurized milk (as contrasted with raw milk) die because of the nutrient loss and other changes in the chemical structure of the milk that pasteurization causes. Experiments have been done in zoos with carnivorous animals. They replaced the raw meat with leftover cooked restaurant meat. The animals in the experiments died. The nutrient loss and structural changes could not support life in these animals.

More animal studies are included under "Enzymes" in Chapter 1 and under "Reproduction" in this chapter.

Reproduction

Francis M. Pottenger, Jr., M.D., along with Alvin Ford, conducted a 10-year "landmark" study starting in 1932. The study was done under the strictest scientific standards. They took approximately nine hundred cats and split them into groups. Six hundred of the cats had complete medical histories. Medical observations were recorded on all of the cats. All the cats were kept outdoors in large pens. The groups had the same conditions except that one group was fed raw milk, raw meat and cod liver oil, while the other group had the same meat, but cooked, pasteurized milk, and the same cod liver oil. The cats fed with raw food (hereafter referred to as 'raw food cats') remained healthy throughout the generations. The cats fed with cooked food (hereafter referred to as 'cooked food cats') were unable to reproduce after the third generation. Therefore, there were no fourth generation cats fed on cooked food to continue the study.

The raw-food cats:
- Were resistant to infections, fleas and parasites.
- Had no changes in skeletal tissue or fur.
- Manifested friendly and predictable mental states.
- Had no trouble birthing or nursing.

The cooked-food cats:
- Were not resistant to infections, fleas and parasites.
- Had unfavorable changes in skeletal tissue and fur.
- Suffered from heart problems, nearsightedness, farsightedness, underactivity or inflammation of the thyroid and bladder, arthritis and inflammation of the joints, inflammation of the nervous system with paralysis and meningitis, and infections of the kidney, bones, liver, testes and ovaries.
- Showed much more irritability than the raw food cats, were unpredictable, bit and scratched. The males had a drop in sexual interest and same-sex sexual activities were observed. (These sexual behaviors were not observed in the raw food cats.)

The symptoms of the cats fed on 100 percent cooked foods sounds very much like those that our society is experiencing today, do they not? Fertility drugs and doctors specializing in fertility are a growing and very profitable business. I believe infertility is mostly related to improper diet and lifestyle choices.

More details on this study can be found in the book, *Pottenger's Cats* by Francis M. Pottenger, Jr., M.D.

Human Studies

In 1950, Dr. Masavore Kuratsuna, head of the Medical Department of the University of Kyushu in Japan, used himself and his wife to validate previous studies comparing the effects of raw and cooked foods on humans. Both of them followed a raw version of the World War II prisoners of war diet that the Japanese had given to their prisoners. It consisted of only 728-826 calories per day: brown rice, vegetables and a little fruit, 22-30 grams of protein, 7.5-8 grams of fat, and 164-207 grams of carbohydrates. They followed a raw version of it for three different periods: 120 days in winter, 81 days in spring and 32 days in summer. During this time, Mrs. Kuratsuna was breast-feeding a baby and found that nursing was less of a strain than before the experiment. Both continued to do their usual work and found themselves in good health. They then switched to eating a cooked version of the same diet. The symptoms of the hunger diseases that devastated the inmates of the Japanese camps, edema, vitamin deficiencies and collapse manifested. They proved that even this inadequate diet could maintain health and even the health of a nursing mother, if eaten raw.

Digestive Leucocytosis

At the Institute of Clinical Chemistry in Lausanne, Switzerland, Paul Kouchakoff did extensive research on digestive leucocytosis. Digestive leucocytosis is the phenomenon of white blood cells (leucocytes) rushing to the intestines as cooked food enters the body.

Before Kouchakoff's work, digestive leucocytosis was thought to be perfectly normal. But Kouchakoff found that when food is eaten raw, digestive leucocytosis does not occur. In fact, he found that if something raw is eaten before something cooked, leucocytosis does not occur.

Jamey Dina, N.D., explains that low temperature cooking may not cause this phenomenon. "The range we have been able to find is between 170 degrees Fahrenheit and 206 degrees Fahrenheit (*Uncooking with Jamey and Kim*)." Dr. Dina's research suggests that keeping your cooking temperature under 170 degrees prevents leucocytosis from occurring.

If one's leucocytes flock to the intestines every time one eats, day after day, the immune system cannot function optimally for the rest of the body. Eating raw foods or low-temperature cooked foods leaves the white blood cells free for other tasks and can only help the body resist disease.

Kirlian Photography

Have you ever been shocked from static electricity? Imagine being able to view a close up picture of that electrical current.

Kirlian photography captures on film the electricity surrounding matter (such as plants and animals). It is not static electricity but a constant field of energy. The picture of the five spheres with tiny lightning bolts shooting from them is a Kirlian photograph of the electrical energy surrounding the author's fingertips (taken in 1990).

I have viewed Kirlian photographs that compare organic and nonorganic foods of the same variety, and in the photos that I have viewed, the organic ones have a superior field of electricity. I have also viewed comparisons of cooked foods versus raw ones, and the raw ones always have a superior field of electricity. David Wolf's book, *Eating for Beauty*, includes these types of photos.

In a comparison of Kirlian photos of human fingertips, I have noticed that people with cleaner diets tend to have larger electrical fields around their fingertips.

Consider what happens to the electrical energy that surrounds living foods after they are eaten. Are we absorbing it and adding it to our own electrical fields? I have no proof of this hypothesis, but I believe that we absorb the electric fields of our foods when we consume them. I believe that this energy is important for our health and gives us greater vitality.

More information can be found at www.kirlian.org.

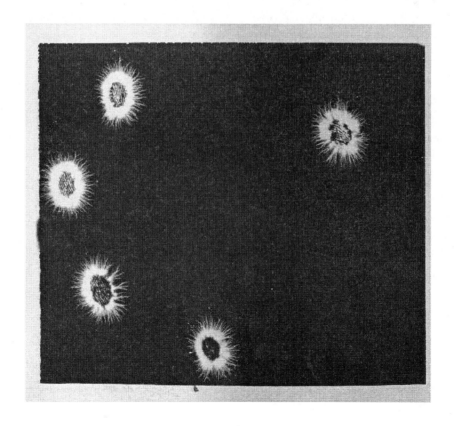

The Mind

A direct connection exists between nutrition and lifestyle choices and the way in which the mind functions. For example, when Vitamin B1 (thiamin) is deficient, depression, irritability, withdrawal, and schizoid tendencies are common symptoms. When Vitamin B3 (niacin) is deficient, anxiety, fatigue, and depression symptoms may occur. Now imagine if all the essential building blocks (foods) and conditions (lifestyle factors) were present. Your mind could function in ways that, for most people, are fleeting. Imagine functioning at your highest potential all of the time.

Professor Arnold Ehret, noted European savant, raw foodist and author of many books, explains how correct nutrition can lead to a state of higher consciousness in his book, *The Mucusless Diet Healing System.*

"If your blood is formed from eating the foods I teach you, your brain will surprise you. Your former life will take on the appearance of a dream and, for the first time in your existence, your consciousness will awaken to a real self-consciousness. Your mind, your thinking, your ideals, your aspirations and your philosophy changes fundamentally in such a way as to beggar description. Your soul will shout for joy and triumph over misery of life, leaving it all behind you. For the first time, you will feel a vibration of vitality through your body (like slight electric current) that shakes you delightfully."

I have experienced exactly what Professor Ehret explains in this quote and believe that most people can experience this transformation as well, if they follow the guidelines in this book.

Robert Ross talks about what it means to be a whole being: "The real value of a whole, raw food diet is that it empowers more than just our health. With a healthy body and healthy mind, we not only think clearly and less reactively, but with greater awareness, understanding, sensitivity and compassion. A healthy, whole being takes full responsibility naturally, doesn't fall into fear and anger with a knee-jerk response to adversity and has compassion for people who seemingly are against us as well as our friends. We have that whole being in us just waiting to come out and all we have to do is stop repressing it with toxic lifestyle and diet choices. Whole raw foods help us get in touch with our natural power. Whole beings are naturally powerful. The toxins in processed and cooked foods, however, block your natural power. Many of these toxins actually have a sedative-like effect on the brain."

Many people claim that while on a living and raw foods diet, they feel more alive and tuned in to themselves, their environments, and others. Some call it a "raw high" to explain how they feel on raw and living foods.

Chapter Three:
Foods for Fuel and Medicine

If you had to depend on an automobile for transportation, and that automobile was designed to run on high octane fuel, would you fill the gas tank with low octane fuel and expect it to perform well? That vehicle would *knock and ping* on a low octane fuel. The same principle applies for humans. If we do not eat the foods that our bodies were designed to run on, we will eventually experience problems in our bodies that you can compare with *knocks, pings, and stalling* of an automobile. My body performs with boundless energy right up until I lie down to sleep at night provided I keep only high quality foods in my diet and don't overeat fats. I believe that I was designed to run on *high octane foods*. If I consume *low octane* (processed) *foods*, my body needs rest to digest them. Some people can get away with consuming *low octane foods* longer than others, depending on their genetics, but it eventually catches up with them and their bodies start to *knock, ping, and stall*.

We cannot expect all foods to have the same effects on all people. Each of us has different nutritional needs and sensitivities. Also note that to get a desired effect from a food we do not need to consume a large or even moderate amount, in some cases less may be more effective than more.

In this chapter we will cover many commonly available foods so that you will understand what *high octane foods* are, how to use foods for medicinal purposes, how to help regulate body temperature with them, and more.

For optimum digestion, use the following chart as a guideline.

Food Combination Chart

Proteins and Fats
Avocado, coconut, nuts, olive,
seeds, beans, yogurt (use nut
yogurt with live cultures)

Mildly Starchy Vegetables
Artichoke, beet, carrot, cauliflower, corn, peas, zucchini
Starches
Pea, potato, sprouted legumes,
squash, sprouted-grain (Essene)
bread, grains, legumes

Poor Combination

Non-Starchy Vegetables
Asparagus, bok choy, broccoli, brussel sprout, cabbage, celery,
chard, collard, cucumber, eggplant, endive, green bean, kale,
lettuce, parsley, spinach, sprouts, peppers, turnip

Good Combination

Use Sparingly
Garlic, leek, onion, radish, scallion, shallot

Good Combination

**Fruits do not combine well with other types of food because they digest more quickly.
Wait at least half an hour after eating fruit before you eat another type of food.**

Sweet Fruits
Bananas, dates, dried
fruits, durian, persimmon,
prune, raisin

Sub-Acid Fruits
Apple, apricot, blueberry,
cherimoya, cherry, fresh
fig, grape, kiwi, mango,
nectarine, papaya, peach,
pear, plum

Acid Fruits
Blackberries, cranberries,
grapefruit, lemon, lime,
orange, pineapple, raspber-
ry, strawberry, tangerine,
tomato

**Melons digest faster than any other food type. Only eat them on an empty
stomach and then wait at least half an hour before eating another type of food.**

Melons
Cantaloupe, casaba,
crane, crenshaw, honey
dew, persian, sharlyn,
watermelon

Fruits and Melons

Ripe fruits are high in vitamins and enzymes and contain ample amounts of phytonutrients, minerals, and amino acids. They are easily digestible and contain super-hydrating purified water. I start each day with fruit as my first meal.

An interesting fact about fruit, and perhaps all natural foods, is that the taste of two identical pieces of fruit can vary greatly, even if the trees that they were picked from were the same varieties and grown side by side in the same conditions! I have experienced this phenomenon many times while blueberry picking. If you have an aversion to a variety of fruit, I encourage you to try it again. Perhaps the last time you tried it you got a bad one.

The following list of fruits and their medicinal qualities is by no means complete. To list all the known fruits and their health benefits would take volumes. In addition, there are numerous varieties of common fruits. For example, more than 1,400 varieties of apples grow around the world. I have listed the fruits that are commonly available in North America and some of the medicinal qualities.

Apples: Canadian scientists found that both unpasteurized fresh apple juice and unpasteurized fresh apple sauce can "knock the heck out of stomach flu and polio virus" (Heinerman p. 4). Apples have been clinically shown to decrease dental cavities and help prevent both diarrhea and constipation. I suggest making your own apple juice and sauce because pasteurization destroys much of their nutritive value.

Avocados: In a study done at the Veteran's. Hospital in Coral Gables, Florida, avocados were shown to lower blood cholesterol. People ranging in age from 27 to 72 years old consumed from ½ to 1¼ avocados per day. Fifty percent showed a definite decrease in serum cholesterol ranging from 8.7 to 42.8 percent (Heinerman p. 16). Research in Israel has shown that eating avocados cut detrimental (LDL) cholesterol about 12 percent in men. These results are thought to be the result of cholesterol-lowering phytosterols that avocados have an abundance of. In South Africa avocados are eaten as an aphrodisiac (Ross p. 243).

Bananas: Plantains are a type of banana that many people fry before eating while the fruit is unripe. The plantain is wonderful eaten raw provided that it is ripe. Ripe plantains are soft and in some varieties the skin needs to turn black before they are edible uncooked. There are numerous varieties of bananas; I seek out the small varieties or the red ones. An interesting medicinal property of the banana is that, "Antifungal and antibiotic principles are found in the peel and pulp of fully ripe bananas. The antibiotic acts against mycobacteria" (Morton p. 45).

Berries: The *Journal of Food Science*, volume 41 (1976) showed that polio virus was inactivated by strawberry extract. Several other fruits such as raspberries, blueberries, and wild cranberries helped to inactivate other intestinal viruses, including herpes simplex virus (Heinerman p. 45). Because of their high potassium content, a major medical journal stated that an extra serving of fresh fruit, such as berries, may decrease the risk of stroke in humans by as much as 40 percent regardless of other known risk factors (Heinerman).

Cherry: The number one remedy for gout is to consume raw cherries. Eat about ½ pound of sweet cherries or drink about 3 tablespoons of cherry juice concentrate per day (spread their consumption out during the day). One also needs to stop consuming foods containing uric acid such as beef, chicken, and other meats to relieve the gout.

Cranberry: These berries prevent unfriendly bacteria from adhering to bladder cells and acidify the urine. Cranberries contain compounds that have antimicrobial activity. They are known best for fighting infections of the urinary tract. More on cranberries under the heading, Berries.

Durian: This football-sized fruit has large spikes protruding from it (picture on front cover) and is available at Asian markets. The smell might put some people off, but the taste is heavenly. Medical anthropologist John Heinerman explains, "Different folk healers with whom I closely worked beat the ripe durian flesh to a juicy pulp and had their patients afflicted with malaria drink and eat this stuff in adequate quantities. I never knew them to fail curing cases of malaria, even when regular prescription drugs failed to eradicate the problem" (Heinerman pg. 135).

Fig: A component of the fruit of the fig tree has been found by a team of Japanese scientists to fight cancer. The July 1978 issue of *Lloydia*, a scientific journal, found that benzaldehyde taken from figs reduced tumors by 39 percent. A subsequent follow-up study with 57 cancer patients showed a 50 percent regression of tumors with the benzaldehyde from figs according to *Cancer Treatment Reports* for January 1980 (Heinerman pg. 144). Figs are also known to be an excellent laxative and a powerful energy-imparting food.

Grapefruit: Dr. James Cerda, professor of gastroenterology at the University of Florida in Gainsville, found that when medium to high-risk patients took 15 grams of grapefruit pectin every day for four months, their serum blood cholesterol levels decreased by almost 10 percent. In 50 percent of the patients tested, the ratio of good to bad cholesterol improved as well. These benefits happened without any other dietary or lifestyle changes (Heinerman pg. 203).

Grapes: In Ottawa Canada, two microbiologists working with the Canadian Health and Welfare Agency discovered that grape juice (probably unpasteurized), raisin tea, and red wine (wine is a raw product) showed strong antiviral activity against polio virus, herpes simplex virus, and reovirus (an apparent cause of meningitis, mild fever, and diarrhea) (Heinerman pg. 209).

Kiwi: The kiwi contains high amounts of potassium and Vitamin C. People looking to lower their blood pressure find that kiwis' high potassium content works well and it's delicious too! Kiwi also contains substantial amounts of Vitamin E and niacin.

Lime: During the seventeen and eighteen-hundreds, the British navy had its sailors eat limes to prevent scurvy, (a fatal disease caused by a Vitamin C deficiency) because of its high Vitamin C content. Some sources claim that the cause of scurvy was known one hundred years before the authorities acknowledged this fact and many sailors may have died needlessly from this preventable disease. This scenario sounds very much like what is happening in modern times. Because of political policies, powerful corporations and other factors related to economics, the public is poorly informed when it comes to proper nutrition.

Lychee: These berries are sometimes mistakenly called nuts. Available in Asian markets, most commonly in the dried form, these berries have a sweet and satisfying taste. Traditional Chinese medicine has used the lychee as a tonic to strengthen the liver and kidneys (which purify the blood) and to improve the performance of the respiratory system in cases of asthma and bronchitis.

Olive: The fruit of the olive tree is high in tannins which makes it very bitter. The tannins are usually removed before eating. There are several methods of removing the tannins. The method that I use when curing olives is an ancient one. The olives are soaked in brine (salt water) for more than a month. By osmosis, most of the tannins are drawn out of the olive into the soak water and then discarded. This method takes a long time, so the commercial olive industry devised a method of curing olives that takes about 3 days. They soak olives in lye (a harsh chemical). This quickly removes the tannins but may leave a residue of lye to be eaten by the consumer. Another factor to be aware of if you are seeking raw olives is that when you purchase olives in jars or cans in the USA they are usually pasteurized (unless they state that they are raw). I buy my olives from a bulk source, such as from five gallon buckets, because they are still raw.

Orange: The human brain has concentrated Vitamin C pumps. The next time you find yourself unable to think clearly, try eating a fresh juicy orange loaded with Vitamin C and bioflavonoids and see if your mind becomes a bit clearer. In China, oranges are used to stimulate digestion, and thus can help alleviate constipation (Ody pg. 48).

Papaya: The seeds of the papaya fruit taste somewhat peppery and make a great substitute for black pepper when ground. They can be used to spice foods or as a medicine to rid the intestinal tract of parasites such as hookworms and roundworms. The fruit pulp of papaya contains an enzyme called papain that is commercially used as a meat tenderizer because it digests protein. John Heinerman explains that papain from papaya is superior to trypsin, and that in animal experimentation, venom from poisonous snakebites was not deadly to animals injected with the enzyme trypsin if the enzyme was administered a short amount of time after the bite. Heinerman says, "...it only stands to reason that it [papain] should be taken orally when an individual is accidentally bitten by a poisonous snake..." (Heinerman pg. 470). Unripe papaya is higher in papain than ripe papaya. Unripe papaya salads are commonly eaten in Thailand, Mexico, and other countries. Although I am a strong believer in eating ripe produce, papaya is the exception to the rule. Papaya is very beneficial to the digestive system because of the papain. When preparing green papaya, be aware that the papain can cause temporary irritation to the skin and should be washed off your hands immediately after preparation.

Passion fruit: Ripe passion fruit will help with insomnia, restlessness, neuralgia, muscle spasms, convulsions, and epilepsy (Heinerman pg. 468).

Peach: This fruit originated in China several thousand years ago. The peach was then known as the fruit of immortality (Heinerman pg. 343).

Persimmon: There are two varieties of persimmons commonly available. The Hachiya is shaped like an acorn and needs to be ripened to the point of having wrinkled skin before it is consumed. The Fuyu is shaped like a tomato and is ready for eating while it is firm. In Thailand the persimmon is used for getting rid of intestinal worms, particularly hookworms (Heinerman pg. 368).

Pineapple: Scientific research has shown that the bromelain found in ripe pineapple can thin human blood and prevent blood clots from forming while increasing circulation (Heinerman pg. 471).

Plums: When dried, the fruit of the plum tree is called a prune. Prunes have long been used as a safe and powerful laxative. Prunes are also high in antioxidants. Be sure to purchase non-sulfured prunes. Sulfur dioxide is commonly used to preserve non-organic dried fruits and may aggravate asthma or have other unwanted side effects.

Pomegranate: This fruit is spoken of with great regard in the Old Testament of the Bible and also by modern researchers. "Pomegranate juice enters into preparations for treating dyspepsia and it is considered beneficial in leprosy." (Morton pg. 355). The seeds are said to expel tapeworm from the intestines. Researchers say that antioxidants are highest in the bright colors of fruits and the pomegranate has bright red juice.

Tamarind: In the West Indies, the fruit pulp is eaten for its laxative properties (*Medicinal Plants of the World* by Ivan A. Ross). In the USA, the pods are usually sold in Asian or specialty food/produce markets. Just peel off the shell of the pod, separate the pulp from the seeds and fibers and eat. The taste is rather pleasant.

Tangerine: Scientific research done in 1965 found that tangerine juice contains an ample amount of synephrine. Synephrine is a well-known decongestant. One glass each morning is suggested to clear mucus out of the lungs (Heinerman pg. 446).

Tomato: The tomato is in fact a fruit and not a vegetable. Vine-ripened and organically grown tomatoes are what we will be discussing here, not genetically modified tomatoes that are picked green, cold-stored for long periods, and gassed with chemicals to achieve a red color. The tomato contains phytonutrients that have been directly linked to the prevention of breast and prostate cancer (*Hippocrates Newsletter* pg. 6). Factory workers in the Soviet Union who have been exposed to toxic chemicals are prescribed tomatoes by doctors to detoxify their livers. There is also some clinical evidence that fresh juice from vine-ripened tomatoes can help the liver regenerate or reproduce a part if another portion has been destroyed or surgically removed (Heinerman pg. 458).

Watermelon and its sprouted seeds: These have diuretic properties and are used to flush the kidneys and bladder (*Hippocrates Newsletter* pg. 6). The rind is high in minerals. Eat watermelon on hot days to reduce body temperature and replace electrolytes lost through sweating.

Vegetables, Roots, Herbs and Spices

In this section, just as in the fruit section, we will cover some of the vegetables commonly available in North America. Almost all vegetables can and should be eaten raw and as freshly harvested as possible. If, however, fresh produce is not available, frozen vegetables are superior to canned vegetables, which I do not recommend.

Basil: There are many types of basil which have different flavors and chemical compositions. In Western folk medicine, basil is used to treat gastrointestinal problems such as stomach cramps and also to treat whooping cough, head colds, headache, and warts. Traditional Chinese medicine uses basil to promote blood circulation, help digestion, and to rid the body of inflammation (Leung pg. 32).

Broccoli: The entire plant is edible, not just the bunches of flowering buds. The leaves are excellent for juicing and the tough stems can be peeled, allowing access to the soft and delicious inner stem. Broccoli has high vitamin content when eaten raw, even higher than carrots. If you are not used to eating raw broccoli, and it gives you gas, fear not. Most people's bodies adapt to eating raw broccoli. Start off slowly with just a sprig and slowly increase your consumption over time. (See cruciferous vegetables for more on broccoli and its anticancer properties.)

Cabbage: Recent clinical trials have demonstrated that cabbage, and especially cabbage juice, is effective for treating stomach ulcers (both gastric and duodenal) (Ody pg. 42). I enjoy making and eating sauerkraut and believe that fermenting the cabbage is more beneficial than consuming it unfermented (see recipe section). (See cruciferous vegetables for more on cabbage.)

Carrot: Many of my clients have told me that after including raw carrots in their daily diet, their night vision improved. I suggest raw carrots as part of a healthy diet. I do not recommend the consumption of carrot juice for those who are suffering from blood sugar problems, cancer, yeast infections, or any bacterial infection. Due to the high sugar content of carrots, their juice has the ability to feed invading pathogens in the same manner as any sugar.

Celery: Traditional Chinese medicine has used celery juice to lower high blood pressure for thousands of years. Celery contains a phytonutrient called phthalide which relaxes smooth muscle tissue that lines artery walls. Celery is an excellent source of organic sodium that has a different effect on us than that of sodium chloride found in table salt. Eating fresh ribs of celery can help stimulate milk flow after childbirth. Although wild celery is more effective, commercially grown varieties can be used (Ody pg. 37). Juicing the whole plant (seeds, root, ribs, and leaves) helps with joint and urinary tract inflammation (Ody pg. 37).

Be certain to ingest only fresh, crisp celery. Once it becomes old and wilted, celery has been found to contain 25 times higher amounts of a chemical called furocoumarin (compared to the tiny amount in fresh celery.) Old celery has caused cancer in animals while fresh celery has not.

Chicory: Egyptian scientists have found that chicory root decreases the rate and volume of heartbeat. This may prove beneficial for treating tachycardia (rapid heartbeat) (Heinerman pg. 108). There are several coffee substitutes that use powdered chicory root and are commonly available in health food stores.

Cruciferous vegetables: Broccoli, brussel sprouts, cabbage cauliflower, kale, and kohlrabi have been found to inhibit the growth of tumors, prevent cancer of the colon and rectum, detoxify the system of harmful chemical additives and increase our body's cancer-fighting compounds. The research has been published in many scientific journals including the *Journal of the National Cancer Institute* (Heinerman pg. 75). These vegetables are high in the mineral sulphur and the phytonutrient sulforaphan which helps fight cancer cells, including the cell growth of breast cancer as reported in the *Journal of Nutrition*.

Corn: The kernels of corn are considered to be nutritive and may stimulate appetite. The silk of the corn has been listed as an official drug in the pharmacopoeia of China for only a few decades. That pharmacopoeia says that corn silk has both diuretic and hypotensive properties and can be used to treat edema, kidney inflammation, urinary difficulties, jaundice, and hypertension.

Cucumber: On a hot day, cucumber is one of the best foods to consume because it is actually able to reduce body temperature after consumption. Herbalists label cucumber a refrigerant. Although cucumbers turn yellow when ripe, green cucumbers (unripe) are healthy.

Daikon radish: This is a Japanese root vegetable that has a long history of assisting the body in blood purification, improved circulation, and the reduction of ulcers (*Hippocrates Newsletter* pg. 5).

Dill seed: Western folk medicine has used dill seed to help the following conditions: lack of appetite, upset stomach, insomnia, and flatulence. Traditional Chinese medicine uses dill seed to treat gastrointestinal problems such as stomachache, vomiting, and lack of appetite (Leung pg. 58).

Endive: This blood builder and liver detoxifier contains a high quantity of minerals and chlorophyll making it similar to nettles and dandelion which are commonly used in the battle to reduce aging and increase vitality (*Hippocrates Newsletter* pg. 5).

Garlic, Onions, and Leeks: Entire books are available that explain all of the health benefits of garlic. In brief, garlic, onions and leaks are naturally antibiotic, antifungal, and antitumor. They lower elevated blood cholesterol and pressure, prevent blood clots, eliminate parasitic worms, and promote healthy circulation. Garlic contains allyl sulfides which researchers believe help to reduce ventricular plaque and inflammation, the cause of both heart attacks and stroke.

Ginger: This root is the most effective antinausea medicine that I am aware of. Ginger promotes blood circulation by thinning the blood. Ginger is a very powerful antioxidant, so I suggest that those searching for eternal youth consume raw ginger every day. It may be added into smoothies, shredded on top of salads, or consumed by drinking homemade ginger tea (slice thin, add to water, steep and drink). Ginger contains a substance called sesquiphellandrene which has been shown helpful to the human body for fighting off the common cold.

Horseradish: A root that has the ability to loosen and remove mucus (expectorant), aid digestion, and possesses anticancer properties.

Kale: Its superior calcium, phosphorous, and magnesium content strengthens the teeth, the skeletal structure, and red blood cells. Its sulphur content assists in the reduction of ulcers and other gastrointestinal disorders (*Hippocrates Journal* pg. 5).

Leek: See garlic.

Lettuces: The leafy green varieties contain a close cousin to opiates which have the ability to heighten positive moods and increase sexual desire (*Hippocrates Newsletter* pg. 5).

Onion: Contains a multitude of phyto-chemicals that help to protect human cells from mutagens, as well as viral, bacterial, and fungal problems. Onions have also been helpful with Lyme's disease. For more on onions, see Garlic.

Oregano: Contains compounds with antimicrobial activity (issue 2520 of New Scientist magazine, 07 October 2005, p. 21). I have used oil of oregano for numerous antimicrobial applications and consider it a powerful medicine.

Peppermint: This common herb which I occasionally add to salads (in very small amounts) has been shown to be very helpful in the treatment of irritable bowel syndrome. For this medicinal purpose, the oil of the plant is consumed inside of enteric-coated capsules. The journal *Phytomedicine* reviewed the evidence of 16 clinical studies, most of them double-blind placebo-controlled crossover studies. The majority of these studies showed a consistent and significant improvement in IBS symptoms. Peppermint increases stomach acidity and aids the body in digestion (Balch and Balch pg. 106).

Turmeric: This root (which resembles ginger) contains a powerful anticancer chemical called curcumin. Researchers have found that curcumin, found in the spice turmeric, interferes with melanoma cells. Tests in laboratory dishes show that curcumin made melanoma skin cancer cells more likely to self-destruct in a process known as apoptosis. The same team of researchers has found that curcumin helped stop the spread of breast cancer tumor cells in the lungs of mice. Turmeric has excellent anti-inflammatory properties also.

Watercress: Western folk medicine uses watercress in the treatment of gout, digestive upsets, cough, tuberculosis, anemia, and catarrh of the upper respiratory tract (Leung pg.170).

Zucchini: This summer squash contains a unique variety of phyto-chemicals that have been noted as protectors of hearing and eyesight. Zucchini also may lessen the severity of PMS. The zucchini flowers provide an extraordinary amount of beta-carotene, one of the most important antioxidants (when consumed in whole foods) for protecting the body from cancer and other invasive diseases (*Hippocrates Newsletter* pg. 6).

Nuts and Seeds

The *Journal of the American Medical Association (JAMA)* reported in the May 27th 1983 issue that Dr. Walter Troll, professor of environmental medicine at the New York University School of Medicine, has found evidence that seems to suggest that plant seeds may lower the risk for developing certain types of cancer generally associated with high meat and fat consumption. Dr. Troll's data from epidemiologic studies indicated that cancers of the breast, prostate, and colon are considerably lower in populations whose diets are rich in 'seed foods'. When mice that were inoculated with melanoma cells were injected with enzymes that occur in seeds, the enzymes prevented the development of cancer. Mice injected with the melanoma cells and not the enzymes developed tumors rapidly (Heinerman pg. 424).

Dr. William Esser ran a fasting and raw food retreat in South Florida from 1950 until the year 2000. He still played tennis and enjoyed good health when he retired in his nineties and had much to say on the topic of nuts. In his book, *The Dictionary of Natural Foods*, Dr. Esser states the following:

"In nutritive value, nuts are superior to any food stuff per pound that we know. It is a common opinion among lay people, as well as medical doctors, that the nut, as a source of protein, is of a low grade and insufficient in supplying the needs of the body in building materials. It is thought that without animal proteins of fish and meat, a high state of health is impossible. This is entirely erroneous. According to scientific investigations carried out by Professor Myer E. Jaffa of the University of California, Prof. F. A. Cajori of Yale University, and Van Slyke, Osborne, Harris and others, the proteins in nuts are superior to those of animal origin."

Dr. Esser also says: "Nut butter made from fresh, raw nuts can be used to the advantage for those who are toothless. Nuts are not difficult to digest when eaten raw and, in proper combination, unsalted. Roasting and broiling in oil at high temperature causes a release of free fatty acids, and the addition of sodium chloride (salt) is sufficient cause for inducing indigestion for even cast iron digestion."

Steer clear of roasted nuts and seeds because the oils that are present in these foods become rancid when heated.

John Harvey Kellogg, M.D., inventor of (you guessed it!) Corn Flakes wrote: "Nuts are free from waste products, uric acid, urea and other tissue wastes which abound in meat. Nuts are aseptic, free from putrefactive bacteria and do not readily undergo decay either in the body or outside of it. Meats, on the other hand, as found in markets, are practically always in an advanced stage of putrefaction. Ordinary fresh dried or salted meats contain from three million to ten times that number of bacteria per ounce, and such meats as hamburger and steak often contain more than a billion putrefactive organisms to the ounce. Nuts are clean and sterile. Nuts are free from trichinae, tapeworm and other parasites, as well as other infections due to specific organisms. Meats are not."

Soaking raw nuts that have brown skins is a good practice if one has the time and is seeking optimum digestion. For example, the skins of almonds contain enzyme inhibitors but these enzyme inhibitors are mostly inactivated when submerged in water for at least six hours. The almonds swell up and become sweeter. Since almond skins are indigestible, I sometimes go one step further and peel the skins. Just place soaked and chilled almonds in very hot tap water for 1 minute. After doing this most almond skins can be removed by pinching the almond between the thumb and forefinger. In the ancient Indian system of Ayurveda, it is recommended to soak almonds. In the United States, raw almonds are pasteurized before reaching the marketplace; they are not technically raw.

Walnuts leave a brownish color to the water after they have been soaked and also taste much better. Nuts without brown skins such as pine nuts and macadamia nuts do not contain enzyme inhibitors, so there is no need to soak them.

Have you ever eaten a raw chestnut? They taste better raw than roasted! I can't figure out why people roast them.

Sesame seeds have been used in traditional Chinese medicine for over 2000 years. They are listed in the Chinese pharmacopeia for the treatment of dizziness, blurred vision, and tinnitus (ringing noise in the ears). Sesame seeds have also been used in the treatment of lack of milk in nursing women and general weakness after an illness (Leung pg.136). They are highly nutritious, especially the black variety which have been used in the treatment of prematurely graying hair. Researchers at Chung Yuan University in Taiwan fed a few tablespoons of ground sesame seeds to people every day for a month. Not only did it significantly lower the subjects' cholesterol (bad LDL cholesterol down 10%) but dramatically improved the antioxidant status of their blood. I consume raw unsalted tahini (sesame seed paste) on a regular basis.

Peanuts are not a nut but a legume. I do not suggest the consumption of peanuts because of the possibility of consuming a mold called aflotoxin. When consumed, aflotoxin must be detoxified by the liver, causing this organ to work overtime. If you do choose to consume peanuts, check each and every one for mold.

Pumpkin seeds are high in zinc, an immune system boosting mineral. Raw pumpkin seeds, well chewed, are effective in driving parasitic worms out of the intestinal tract. I say, "A handful of raw pumpkin seeds a day helps keep the doctor away."

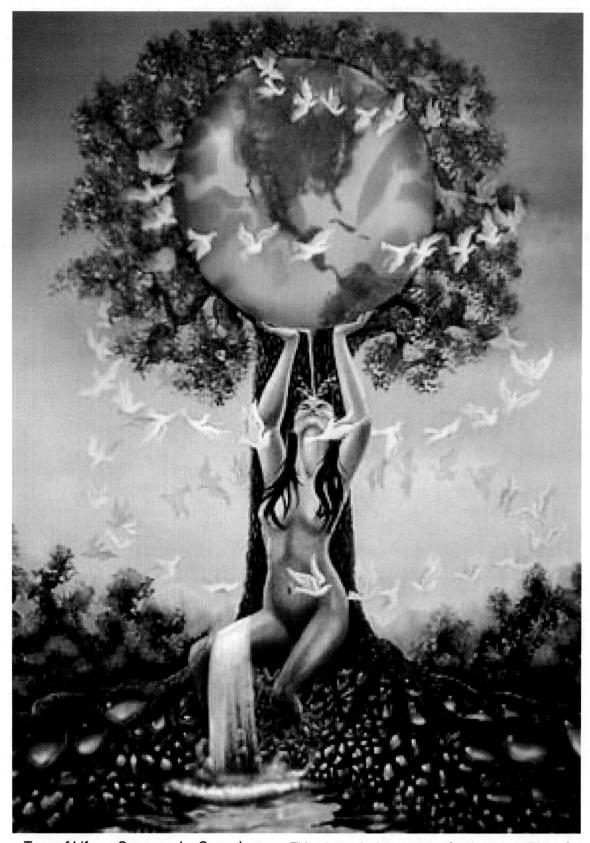

Tree of Life – Summer, by Gwen Ingram. This picture is the cover art for the new edition of

"The Destiny of Women" by Guru Rattana, Ph.D. -available from http://www.yogatech.com

The Nutrient Data Table on the following p. is reprinted from *The Cracker*, January 2000, published by the International Tree Nut Council.

Nutrients in 100 Grams of Tree Nuts

Nutrient	Units	Almond	Cashew	Hazelnut	Macadamia	Pecan	Pistachio	Walnut
Calories	Kca	578	574	628	716	691	567	654
Protein	G	21	15	15	8	9	21	15
Total Fat	G	51	46	61	76	72	46	65
Carbohydrate	G	20	33	17	13	14	27	14
Fiber	G	12	3	10	8	10	10	7
Sugars	Mg	5	NA	4	4	4	8	3
Calcium	Mg	248	45	114	70	70	108	104
Iron	Mg	4	6	5	3	3	4	3
Magnesium	Mg	295	260	163	118	121	120	158
Phosphorus	Mg	474	490	290	196	277	485	346
Potassium	Mg	728	565	680	363	410	1033	441
Sodium	Mg	1	16	0	5	0	1	2
Zinc	Mg	3	6	2	1	5	2	3
Copper	Mg	1	2	2	1	1	1	2
Manganese	Mg	3	1	6	3	4	1	3
Selenium	Mc	8	12	4	4	6	8	5
Vitamin C	Mg	0	0	6	1	1	2	1
Thiamin	Mg	0.2	0.2	0.6	0.7	0.7	0.8	0.3
Riboflavin	Mg	0.8	0.2	0.1	0.1	0.1	0.1	0.1
Niacin	Mg	4	1	2	2	1	1	2
Pantothenic Acid	Mg	0	1	1	1	1	1	
Vitamin B6	Mg	0.1	0.3	0.6	0.4	0.2	1.7	0.5
Folate	Mc	29	69	113	10	22	50	98
Vitamin B12	Mc	0	0	0	0	0	0	0
Vitamin A	IU	10	0	40	0	77	533	41
Vitamin E	Mg	26	1	15	1	4	4	3
Saturated Fat	G	4	9	4	12	6	4	6
Monounsaturated	G	32	27	46	59	41	25	9
Polyunsaturated	G	12	8	8	1	22	14	47
Linoleic Acid	G	12	8	8	1	21	14	38
Linolenic Acid	G	0	0	0	0	1	0	9
Phytosterols	G	120	158	96	114	102	214	72
Cholesterol	**Mg**	**0**	**0**	**0**	**0**	**0**	**0**	**0**

(NA = Not Available)

Sprouts

Most sprouts are easily digestible because of their high content of available enzymes and because the sprouting process predigests the nutrients of the seed. Tests have shown that when seeds are sprouted, their nutrient content increases by 50 to 400 percent (Rita Romano, *Dining in the Raw*). Sprouts have 10 to 30 times more nutrients than the vegetables that they grow into.

That's not all. Sprouting a grain like wheat turns it from an acid- forming food into an alkaline-forming one. To see why this is important, refer to "Acid/ Alkaline Balancing" in chapter 7.

Sprouting is as easy as 1-2-3:

- Soak your seeds in pure water for about 8 hours (except buckwheat).
- Drain the water off the seeds and rinse them 2 to 3 times daily.
- Harvest the sprouts when they grow roots!

Most sprouts can be grown in the dark but darkness is not necessary. The leafy ones like alfalfa need daylight to become green. Once the sprouts are mature, store them in the refrigerator, in a breathable container they are alive and need to breathe. Rinse once every three days but, ideally, eat as soon as possible. Buckwheat needs only two hours to soak and must be rinsed frequently. If soaked longer they may become slimy. Buckwheat is not suggested for those new to sprouting.

I have been sprouting all types of greens and grains in my camper for years, which leads me to believe that it can be done almost anywhere, by anyone.

I personally do not eat sprouted beans often because they sometimes create gas in my system. I refrain from eating alfalfa sprouts because they are said to contain a substance called carayanine which is suspected of causing adverse effects on the health of some people. I also avoid eating buckwheat greens (sprouted buckwheat seeds do not seem to be a problem) because of a naturally occurring substance called fagopyrin occurring in the green leaf. This substance is known to cause hypersensitivity to sunlight in animals and some people. Fagopyrin can cause the skin to turn red or pink and develop a burning sensation when exposed to the sun. I do eat sprouted kamut (an unhybridized strain of wheat).

Other sprouts that agree with me and I enjoy eating include clover, fenugreek, mustard, broccoli, radish, lentil, onion and sunflower in reasonable quantities. I use some of these sprouts to spice my food rather than using dried spices that have lost much of their nutritional value and vibrancy.

Green Foods

The healing power of green foods is extraordinary. Chlorophyll is the substance that gives green plants their color. Hemoglobin, also known as red cells, in human blood and chlorophyll, the blood of the plant, are very similar. They have similar atoms grouped around an atom of metal. The only difference is that the metallic atom in hemoglobin is iron while in chlorophyll it is magnesium. Thus chlorophyll is an excellent source of magnesium. This may explain why chlorophyll has the power to build human blood and increase the oxygen-carrying capacity of our blood.

Disease-promoting anaerobic bacteria cannot live in the presence of oxygen. So as we ingest chlorophyll-rich foods, we can super-oxygenate our bodies and fight off the anaerobic bacteria. Chlorophyll has been successfully used for deodorization and has the power to destroy bad breath that emanates from the stomach. It is commonly sold in health food stores for that purpose and has been used with success for high blood pressure, anemia, and some stomach ailments.

A juicer is an easy way to get large amounts of chlorophyll into your body fast; some sources say it can be assimilated in 20 to 30 minutes. "Green juices cleanse the body of pollutants and have a rejuvenating effect. Made from a variety of green vegetables, green juices are rich in chlorophyll, which helps to purify the blood, build red blood cells, detoxify and heal the body, and provide the body with fast energy." (Balch and Balch pg. 717)

My favorite sources of chlorophyll are common salad greens such as romaine lettuce, bok choy, parsley, and kale. There is a wide variety of gourmet greens to choose from in most supermarkets and especially Asian markets such as mizuna, tat soi, baby lettuces of many varieties and green spices such as basil. I also enjoy concentrated sources such as barley green powder and chlorella, available at health food stores. Whether you get it through juicing leafy greens or wheatgrass, eating green salads, mixing up green powders, or popping green pills, get your daily dose of chlorophyll for a healthy, clean smelling body!

Grains

When wheat is processed to become white flour, it has at least twenty-five **known** nutrients removed from it in the refining process. Yet, it is fortified with only five. These five added nutrients are B1 (thiamine), B2 (riboflavin), B3 (niacin), folic acid and iron. The wheat grown today has been hybridized and is very different from the wheat grown during the Bronze Age. This difference might explain why wheat allergies are so widespread.

Of all the grains, wheat causes the most allergic reactions. Gluten comprises approximately 78 percent of the total protein in modern wheat, and gluten contains an intestinal irritant called gliadin. Gluten is hidden in a very large percentage of processed foods. In addition to wheat, rye, barley, spelt, kamut, and triticale also contain gluten. It is the gluten in flour that causes many wheat allergies (from moderate to severe), and it is also gluten that gives wheat flour its glue-like properties. In fact, children are often given white flour to mix with water to make glue because it dries hard and stiff. However, if you do the same with whole-wheat flour, it will not dry hard nor will it function as glue. Thus white four is a major cause of constipation.

Celiac Sprue is the name given to the condition of severe gluten intolerance. The most common symptom is gastrointestinal distress such as gas, abdominal pain, and diarrhea. The harder to associate symptoms include anemia, depression, fatigue, joint pain, headaches (including migraines), infertility, skin rashes, lactose intolerance, stunted growth in children, schizophrenia, and weight loss (caused by the inability to absorb nutrients). For in-depth lists of gluten containing foods, contact the Celiac Sprue Association/USA at www.csaceliacs.org, or the Celiac Disease Foundation at www.celiac.org. For in-depth information on gluten sensitivity, the book *Dangerous Grains* by James Braly, M.D. and Ron Hoggan, M.A. is very informative.

Amaranth is spoken of in the Eat the Weeds section.

Kamut is a good alternative to the more common types of wheat (including soft and hard red winter wheat). Because kamut is an ancient unhybridized form of wheat, many people who are intolerant of modern hybridized species do not react to kamut (people with celiac disease cannot tolerate kamut). Kamut contains approximately 40 percent more protein than modern wheat and has all 8 essential amino acids. In the Recipes section, you can find directions on how to make Essene bread (sprouted grain bread) from kamut.

Millet can safely be consumed by those with celiac disease because it is completely free of gluten.

Oats are steamed before going to market unless you purchase oat groats for sprouting. Oats are the only grain that is almost always sold as a one hundred percent whole grain. If you find yourself at a restaurant craving a grain, order oatmeal to be sure you're getting a whole grain food. It is also easy to enjoy oatmeal without cooking. Soak a bowl of "slow cook" (as opposed to instant, which is more processed) oats in the refrigerator or, if your house is not too warm, the counter overnight. In the morning, you will have delicious oatmeal with a similar consistency as if it had been cooked. Many people have told me that they did not like oatmeal but found soaked oatmeal to be enjoyable. In reference to oats, the American Heart Association states that it, "Meets American Heart Association food criteria for saturated fat and cholesterol for healthy people over age two." The fact that cholesterol is manufactured in the liver of animals, and all plants are free of cholesterol, makes this an amusing statement to me.

Though both rolled oats and wild rice have been steamed before they go to market and are no longer living foods, they are still far superior to wheat flour products like bread and pasta.

Quinoa (pronounced keen-whah) is perhaps the most amazing grain of all. The World Health Organization states that this South American native is a complete protein with an amino acid profile similar to that of, and at least equal to, cow's milk. It is 16 percent protein (more than any other grain), a good source of minerals and contains more calcium than cow's milk. It is a good source of B vitamins, Vitamin E, iron and phosphorus. Quinoa helps to alkalinize the body. It is also said to be very easy to digest, an important factor for nutrient absorption. This grain is also easy to sprout. Soak it overnight, drain the water and rinse it 3 times per day. Usually within 48 hours it will be ready and tiny tails will be visible. I enjoy eating quinoa sprouted with some extra-virgin olive oil and raw apple cider vinegar. Some people find it too chewy this way, but others love it! Quinoa comes in a variety of colors and I understand that there are approximately 1000 varieties.

Spelt is similar to kamut and is my second choice in grains if kamut is not available.

Teff has a high concentration of nutrients. This grain is very high in calcium and contains high levels of phosphorus, copper and iron. The iron from teff is easily absorbed by the body. Teff is high in protein. It is considered to have an excellent amino acid composition (including all 8 essential amino acids for humans) and has higher lysine levels than wheat or barley. Teff is said to stimulate the flora of the large intestine and is high in carbohydrates and fiber. It contains no gluten, so it is appropriate for those with gluten intolerance or Celiac disease.

Wild rice is always steamed before going to market. It is a grain that can be eaten without further cooking. One must first soak it until some of the grains split down the middle. Soaking time varies on the batch and can take from overnight to several days. (I even had a batch once that never split.) You should change the water daily. I soak my rice in the refrigerator after the first day. After some or most grains have split open, I add apple cider vinegar, olive oil and chopped red peppers to make a nice dish. I should note here that the texture of soaked rice is chewier than cooked rice and can be too tough for people with very bad teeth.

Tea

In China, it is widely believed that green tea is a source of Vitamin C. Since Vitamin C is destroyed by heat, we are left with the question, "Is this belief valid?" According to Kit Chow and Ione Kramer in the book, *All the Tea in China*, research was done in China on the medicinal properties of teas. "Heat destruction does occur, but not in tea (green tea). Something, as yet undetermined, apparently helps stabilize Vitamin C." Is it because green tea contains powerful antioxidants called polyphenols? Green tea has been shown to combat stomach and skin cancers, and to boost the immune system (Ody pg. 44).

The amount of Vitamin C varies greatly depending on growing conditions, the age of the leaves at picking time, and how long they have been stored. Japanese tests found that tea stored three years had lost all its Vitamin C.

As for black tea, authorities have long believed that almost all its Vitamin C is destroyed during fermentation. The fermentation process intensifies the stimulant properties of the tea leaves. Tannins found in tea reduce iron absorption. Mineral analyses in my clinical practice have shown that black tea drinkers accumulate high levels of the toxic mineral cadmium. I do not recommend black tea for anyone and especially those with stomach ulcers or acid reflux because black tea can stimulate gastric acid production.

While traveling in Asia, I visited a tea plantation. Immediately upon entering the building where the black tea is fermented, I became nauseated from the odor released from the fermentation process. I haven't been nauseated by anything since, or for as many years as I can remember before that.

Regarding herbal teas, some, such as roots and barks, need longer heating times. Others, such as flowers and leaves can have their medicinal properties destroyed by boiling and do not need to be heated for much time at all.

For leaves and flowers, I believe the infusion method is best. Place your herbs in a strainer lined with a nonbleached coffee filter. Place the strainer on top of a bowl and pour very hot water (not boiled) over the herbs. What fills your bowl will be the herbal tea.

For roots, barks, berries, nuts and seeds, I feel that the decoction method works best. Soak the herbs in distilled water overnight to soften them and then simmer in a covered pot for at least 15 minutes. Strain and drink!

Brigitte Mars contributed the following information on cold water infusions. "The following flowers make delicious sun teas, without the use of any heat. Fill a glass pitcher with fresh flowers (1 cup flowers to 1 gallon water) from the list that follows. Cover with pure water. Allow to steep in the sun (or moonlight) for several hours. Strain and imbibe the beauty of fresh flower infusions! The infusion will keep up to four days in the refrigerator." I often enjoy Sun Tea and I hope you will also!

Anise hyssop leaf and flower (Agastache foeniculum)
Bee balm leaf and flower (Monarda species)
Catnip leaf and flower (Nepeta cataria)
Lavender flower (Lavandula species)
Lilac flower (Syringa species)
Lemon balm leaf and flower (Melissa officinalis)
Lemon verbena leaf (Aloysia triphylla)
Peppermint leaf and flower (Mentha piperita)
Rose flower and hip (Rosa species)
Rosemary leaf and flower (Rosmarinus officinalis)
Spearmint leaf and flower (Mentha spicata)

Sea Salt

I would like to clarify the difference between iodized/kosher table salt and unprocessed sea salt. To do this, I quote Donna Gates, author of *The Body Ecology Diet*. "We haven't been eating salt in this country. We have been eating this stuff in a blue cardboard box that has a little girl with an umbrella on it, and that's not really salt. In order to make that stuff, they took salt and refined all the minerals out of it, they put in sugar, bicarbonate of soda and lots of other chemicals. They really honestly should not be allowed to call that stuff salt. It confused millions of Americans for generations and generations into thinking that they were eating salt. Then we ran into problems with blood pressure."

Iodized table salt has had all the minerals removed by processing that uses chemicals such as sulfuric acid, chlorine, and hydrochloric acid. The salt is then heated to temperatures around 400 degrees to dry it completely. Usage of this type of salt can lead to excess iodine buildup in the body and impair thyroid function. But unprocessed sea salt has numerous minerals including iodine (not just sodium and iodine) and when consumed in moderation, does not throw the body out of balance.

Unprocessed sea salt, such as Celtic brand hand-harvested sun-dried sea salt, clumps together and does not work in a saltshaker. This type of salt is either pinched out or used in a salt grinder (similar to a pepper grinder). When a salt grinder is not available, I soak the hard salt crystals in a small amount of water and then pour the water on my food. This is the only type of salt that I recommend. There are several companies that package unprocessed sea salt other than Celtic brand. I harvest and sun-dry my own sea salt, but that's a topic for another book.

Most health food stores sell sea salt that has anticaking agents and is less processed than iodized table salt. I suggest going for the better unprocessed salts. They cost a little more but are worth it because of their heath benefits and their wonderful flavor! Real unprocessed salt is very alkalinizing to the tissues and loaded with trace minerals. But don't overdo it; use this food in very small amounts.

Ocean-Grown Food

Readers Digest, August 2003, printed an article called, "Hidden Dangers In 'Healthy' Foods" revealing startling news. The following is an excerpt from the article. "Many Americans are ingesting potentially dangerous levels of mercury by eating store-bought fish - gleaming, fresh, healthy-looking fish that they thought was good for them. Hightower's [Internist Jane Hightower] findings have triggered a furor at the highest levels of the federal government, convinced California to post warnings at fish counters, and stirred fears that something in our diet may be connected to mushrooming rates of learning disabilities. Today, nearly every state has issued warnings about mercury in fish. According to the article, many fish have, on occasion, been recorded as having unsafe levels of mercury. The worst are swordfish, mackerel, marlin, shark, king and tilefish. The second worst are tuna, trout, red snapper, flounder, freshwater bass, grouper and halibut." Fish and shellfish also carry a high risk for many food-borne bacterial illnesses like salmonella. (For further information, refer to "Food-Borne Illnesses" in Chapter 7.)

Because mercury is excreted through breast milk and the chance of lowering a child's IQ increases as the mother's blood-mercury level rises, I caution strongly against the consumption of fish by pregnant women and nursing mothers. A much safer way to get the nutrients that are in fish without the risks involved in eating fish meat is to eat lower on the food chain; in other words, eat sea vegetables.

Humans have a history of eating sea vegetables (seaweeds) dating back thousands of years. Sea vegetables were, and still are, known for their ability to prolong life, prevent disease, and impart beauty and health. Sea vegetables were not just eaten in the Asian countries; the Scots and the Britons used dulse and Irish moss as well.

The nutrient profile of sea vegetables is very impressive. Compared to land plants, they contain **10 to 20 times the mineral content** (including calcium, iodine and iron), are high in protein and have an abundance of vitamins and fiber. Sea vegetables are very low in calories and fat which makes them an excellent food for those who wish to lose weight.

The seaweeds hijiki, arame, and wakame have been analyzed in their dried state. Each contains more than ten times the calcium of cow's milk. Hijiki contains eight times the iron in beef, and wakame and kelp have about four times the iron in beef. Kelp, kombu and arame contain 100 – 500 times the iodine in marine fish. One hundred grams of nori contains 35.6 grams of protein. Arame and hijiki are rich in vitamins and niacin (*Natural Awakenings*, January, 2003 by Jan London). In addition, seaweeds contain alginic acid, a polysaccharide compound that has the ability to chelate (bind compounds to remove them from the body) heavy metals like lead and radioactive elements, as well as excessive sodium (*The New Whole Food Encyclopedia* by Rebecca Wood, p. 360).

The most common sea veggies eaten raw, right out of the package, are dulse, kelp and nori. Most people find dulse delicious as it melts in your mouth! All types of sea veggies may be eaten without cooking; you can soak them for easier digestion and to improve the texture and taste. When I visit pristine waters, such as the Monterey Bay National Marine Sanctuary in California, I eat the sea vegetables directly out of the ocean with only a salt water rinse. I have learned that if the seaweed is growing in shallow waters, and you pick it from its growing place, it is edible. The only non-edible seaweeds are those that grow in deep waters. So don't eat seaweed that has washed up on the beach unless you can identify it. I can harvest enough seaweed in one day to last me an entire year. I sun-dry it and store it in airtight bags when fully dry.

Certain fish, such as tuna, are found to be high in the toxic metal mercury, and can cause a toxic buildup in humans when eaten. Shellfish filter large amounts of water, absorbing bacteria, viruses, and natural toxins, such as heavy metals and chemical contaminants. These creatures, especially oysters, clams and mussels, can cause mild to severe cases of food poisoning when consumed if they are contaminated. Shellfish can also become contaminated with salmonella and/or campylobacter bacteria, either from fecal pollution of water or from improper processing or preparation. Sea vegetables, however, do not absorb these toxins like the filter feeders, which makes them much safer than sea animals. (*Natural Awakenings*, January 2003, Jan London).

Eat the Weeds

When most people look at a lawn full of dandelions they see weeds. I see powerful medicine and nutritious food! Dandelion has many medicinal qualities; it is a blood and liver cleanser, a diuretic, it increases bile production, reduces serum cholesterol and uric acid levels, improves functioning of the kidneys and pancreas, spleen, and stomach, and has many other benefits! (Look it up in a good medicinal herb book!) Dandelion is high in beta carotene, lutein, Vitamins B1, B2, B3, and C, and the minerals calcium, magnesium, iron, manganese, potassium, selenium, and zinc. Many of the plants that grow in your own back yard and in vacant lots are edible and highly nutritious. Yet most people go out to the store and spend their money on iceberg lettuce that is very low in nutrition. Why? Probably it is because they were never taught how or why to eat the native plants. I asked my friend Frank Cook who is a graduate of the Northeast School of Botanical Medicine (1995) to say a few words on weeds. Here is what he said.

"Perhaps you have come to see the weeds as your friends, but it is still a belief by many peoples that weeds are bad and should be eradicated by any means possible. There are many weeds that you can use for food, teas or medicine and for other basic needs as well. Weeds also occupy niches in complex ways that we are only beginning to understand.

"The majority of Americans consume only a couple of dozen plant species in their diet, yet a few hundred years back, the inhabitants of this land consumed over 200 kinds of plants in their diets. This change seems to be at the root of our alienation from the earth.

"I could rattle off the impressive figures of how weeds feed us in macronutrient ways, but it would take up volumes. We are told that we use only 10 percent of our brain capacity. Maybe all those neurons that we don't currently use need the nutrients hidden in the weeds! Weeds have been here with us since we came to be. They shaped and formed us.

"Get to know the weeds beneath your feet. Get your hands on some good weed books, such as *Botany in a Day*, by Thomas Elpels, which teaches you to recognize plant families. Know a dozen plant families and you will recognize over 75 percent of the plants that you meet!

"I want to encourage you to nibble the plants that you are getting to know! As you move about through each day, reach out and touch, smell, admire, and yes, certainly taste those plants which you have come to know as friends. It can be demonstrated that by nibbling weeds, we obtain numerous micronutrients and catalysts. I personally nibble on plants throughout the day and find that it helps me to ground and center and acclimate to the setting I am in, because I travel a lot.

"The names of the most common plant families are: asteraceae pea, buckwheat, grass, mustard, mint, parsley, goosefoot and lily. Learn them first; you will see them around your garden. Learn from and share with others. Grow to know them and you will always be fed! They are waiting to meet you. Learn them! Nibble them!"

Brigitte Mars is a well known herbalist and author. You can read more about her in the "Noteworthy People" section of this book. She has contributed the following article on wild foods which includes gathering guidelines and some extraordinary wild edible plants and flowers!

"Thirty-some years ago I lived in a tipi on a commune in Reynolds, Missouri. There I learned from the local hills people that most of the weeds pulled from gardens were useful edible plants. Rather than composting these so called "weeds," we would incorporate them in meals and thus double or triple the yield of our garden.

Wild foods are hardy. They survive without fertilizer or weekly waterings from the garden hose. Some, like dandelions, continue to survive despite many attempts to get rid of them! Their ability to overcome all sorts of adversity can impart to us humans a source of strength and versatility. Wild things can furnish more nutrition than their cultivated progeny. These are plants nourished by rain, sunlight, moonlight, and wind. Learn to enjoy the freshness of a salad that was collected five minutes before being eaten! Or even eat some wild plants in nature just fresh seconds after gratefully plucking a few parts. Love the weeds that heal and feed our needs!"

Gathering Guidelines:

*Make sure you are collecting the proper species, because many plants have poisonous lookalikes. Bring along a good guide or a good guidebook.

*Be sure you are collecting the correct plant part. For example, blue elderberries are wonderful, but the leaves of the plant are toxic.

*Do not harvest any known endangered species.

*Ask permission before gathering on private land.

*If possible, water plants the day before collecting.

*When harvesting from a group of plants, identify the grandfather/mother plant and leave it to ensure the continuation of the strongest of the species.

*Never take more than 10 percent of a wild population of plants. Leave some for the wild animals!

*Vary the places you collect from.

*Avoid collecting plants within 50 feet of a busy road or in areas that are polluted or have been treated with pesticides or herbicides.

*Gather leaves and flowers in the morning, after the dew has risen and before the sun is too hot.

*Gather leaves not when the plant is already flowering but before, when its energy will still be in its leaves.

*It is kinder to take a whole leaf rather than tearing a leaf.

*Replant seeds as often as possible.

*Collect plants in a way as to ensure the continued survival of the species. For example, if all you need are the leaves and flowers, take only the tops. Cutting a plant back can actually help to promote new growth. Leave the roots to continue their growing cycle. Also help thin plants growing too close together to help the other plants have more room.

*Compost herb parts you do not eat, or use them as mulch or in herbal preparations.

*Sing while collecting! Be joyful!

Amaranth (*Amaranthus* species) Parts used: Leaf and seed. Amaranth, also known as pigweed or redroot, is so persistent that the Greeks considered it a symbol of immortality. Amaranth leaves can be collected before flowering and eaten raw like spinach. The seeds can be collected in late summer or autumn, spread out on a paper bag, and allowed to dry for several days. Using your fingers, separate the seeds from the chaff and use a colander to separate the two. The seeds then can be ground or used as flour and added to dehydrated breads. Amaranth leaves are considered astringent and diuretic. Amaranth leaf tea has been utilized to treat diarrhea, dysentery, and excessive menstrual bleeding. Amaranth does contain some oxalates, which can inhibit calcium absorption, so be sure your diet contains calcium if incorporating more than small amounts of amaranth.

Chickweed (*Stellaria media*) Parts used: Leaf, flower, and stem. More than thirty bird species, including chickens, are known to eat this plant. Chickweed actually makes an excellent ground cover, as it grows outward instead of upward. Its very presence indicates a fertile soil, and it helps the soil retain its nitrogen content. Chickweed is delicate and delicious. The leaves, flowers and stems can be included in salads or made into soups. It keeps well in the refrigerator for up to a couple of weeks. Chickweed is known for its high Vitamin C content. Traditionally, it has been used to strengthen frail people. It has soothing and anti-inflammatory properties and can be prepared as a tea for bladder irritation, bronchial irritation and ulcers. It is an excellent salve ingredient, helping to soothe everything from diaper rash to psoriasis.

Dandelion (*Taraxacum officinale*) Parts used: Leaf, flower, and root. Though most people regard this plant as a nuisance, dandelion is rich in uses. The leaves are edible, and taste better in the springtime, before the plant flowers, and are high in iron and beta-carotene. The leaves also have a diuretic effect. Most chemical diuretics deplete the body of potassium, but dandelion greens, in contrast, are rich in this mineral. Dandelion blossoms can be separated from the calyx and sprinkled on salads. They contain lutein, a nutrient beneficial for the eyes. Dandelion roots also are edible. We like to dig them up, scrub them, add a bit of olive oil and Nama Shoyu, and then dehydrate them a bit. Delicious! Dandelion root tea has long been used to improve skin conditions such as acne and eczema and improves liver function.

Knotweed (*Polygonum erectum, P. aviculare*) Parts used: Above ground plant and seed. Knotweed, also known as doormat grass, is considered an important kidney herb; it is a valuable diuretic and can be used to eliminate kidney stones. The genus name is derived from the Greek polys, meaning 'many', and gony, meaning 'knees', in reference to the many jointed stems of the plant. This is perhaps what led knotweed to be used as a tea remedy for swollen arthritic joints and knees. Its high silica content makes it a good remedy for strengthening the lungs' connective tissue. When knotweed stems are young and tender, between 6 to 8 inches in height, they can be collected, chopped fine and added to salads. The seeds can also be collected and used as a grain.

Lambsquarter (*Chenopodium album*) Parts used: Leaf and seed. The goosefoot-shaped leaves of this abundant plant have long been used as a nourishing food during times of war and famine. The leaves taste like spinach but are much easier to grow and are even more nutritious. Being rich in iron, lambsquarter is considered a remedy for anemia. The seeds can also be collected and used as a grain.

Malva (*Malva neglecta*) Parts used: Leaf, flower, and seed. Malva leaves are soothing and anti-inflammatory. They can be eaten by themselves or added to soups; their rich mucilage content helps thicken the pot's contents. Made into a tea, malva leaves are a traditional medicine for sore throats and ulcers. They also make a simple poultice for treating skin rashes, burns and insect bites. The leaves are very rich in beta carotene and have been included in teas and syrups for helping coughs and irritated lung conditions. The delicate pink and white flowers are a lovely and edible addition to grace the dinner plate. The seeds are edible and can be eaten raw or even pickled. The seeds have a high moisture content; when water is scarce, they can be used to moisten the mouth.

Mustard (*Alliaria petiolata, A. officinalis, Brassica juncea, B. sinapiodes, Cardaria draba, Descurania species, Lepidium perfoliatum, Sinapsis alba, Sisymbrium officinale*) Parts used: Leaf, seed, seedpod, and flower. Mustard is an annual growing from 1 to 8 feet in height, depending on the species. Mustard flowers range in color from white, pink, yellow, and purple, but all have four petals in the shape of a cross with four sepals, six stamens and one pistil. Both the seeds and leaves are used as food and medicine. Mustard is considered antiseptic, expectorant, rubifacient and stimulant. It has been used medicinally to treat chilblains, cough, and respiratory congestion. Mustard stimulates appetite and gastric juices. Its qualities are pungent and hot. Leaves can be chopped and mixed with other milder greens in a salad. Flowers are edible in salads and as a garnish. Young seedpods are also edible. Seeds are used in pungent sauces. There are no poisonous mustards, however, eat only in moderation as mustards do contain some irritating oils that can cause intestinal irritation.

Nettles (*Urtica dioica*) Part used: Young plant. Nettles are probably best known for their sting. The tiny hairs of the plant contain formic acid, the same stinging substance that causes pain from ant bites. The hairs also contain choline acetyltransferase, acetlylcholine, choline, and serotonin. There are actually health benefits to the stings, such as in relieving arthritis pain. Most people will want to wear gloves and use scissors when collecting nettles. However, people in the know have learned that getting stung by nettles is very therapeutic and relieves pain and inflammation. I have several friends that "whack" their wrists in the nettle patch to relieve the soreness from playing guitar all night long. Young nettles shoots can be finely chopped and marinated in a bit of olive oil, Celtic salt, and lemon juice. Nettles can also be pureed in a food processor to make a pesto. (Pureeing them deactivates the sting.) Nettles are highly alkaline and very rich in iron; they are more effective than spinach in building the blood. Their rich supply of beta carotene and Vitamin C strengthens the mucus membranes. In fact, nettles are so rich in nutrients that they help curb overeating. Nettles also are considered anti-allergenic. Taking nettles in capsule, tea or tincture form before the hay fever season even begins can minimize the annual discomfort of hay fever. Only young nettles plants should be consumed; once the plant starts to flower, it becomes irritating to the kidneys when ingested.

Purslane (*Portulaca oleracea*) Part used: Leaf. Though its creeping succulent leaves seem tenacious invaders, purslane is truly a valuable plant. It is rich in omega-3 fatty acids and helpful in protecting the heart and lowering blood pressure and cholesterol levels. It is a cooling summer vegetable rich in beta carotene and Vitamin C. Not only does it make a fine salad herb, but is wonderful in raw soups like gazpacho.

Violet (*Viola odorata*) Parts used: Leaf and flower. As we look deep into shady areas, heart-shaped leaves and brilliant purple flowers announce the ever-present violet. You might catch its beautiful aroma before you glimpse it. Violet leaves are wonderful in salads. The flowers are in their prime in the spring. The leaves and flowers are both high in Vitamin C and an esteemed remedy for coughs, fevers and lung complaints such as bronchitis. The smell and flavor of violets is said to help comfort one who is grief stricken.

Flowers, the sex organs of plants, add grace and beauty to any dish you make and are a wonderful addition to a raw foods diet. Be sure to use only organically grown or wild edible flowers, as many commercial ones are treated with chemicals.

The following chart of edible flowers has been provided by Brigitte Mars. For most flowers do not eat the center, only the petals.

Acacia (Acacia species)	Marigold (Tagetes erecta, T. tenufolia)
Anchusa (Anchusa officinalis, A. azurea)	Marjoram (Origanum marjorana)
Anise hyssop (Agastache foeniculum)	Meadowsweet (Filipendula ulmaria)
Apple blossoms (Malus species)	Mint (Mentha species)
Arugula (Eruca sativa)	Mullein (Verbascum species)
Bachelor's buttons (Centaurea cyanus)	Mustard (Brassica species)
Banana (Musa species)	Nasturtium (Tropaeolum majus)
Basil (Ocimum basilicum)	Okra (Abelmoschus esculentus)
Bee balm (Monarda species)	Onion (Allium species)
Begonia (Hybrid tuberous begonia)	Orange blossom (Citrus sinensis)
Borage (Borago officinalis)	Oregano (Origanum species)
Broccoli (Brassica oleracea)	Pansy (Viola wittrockiana)
Calendula (Calendula officinalis)	Passionflower (Passiflora species)
Canary creeper (Tropaeolum peregrinum)	Pea (Pisum sativum)
Carnation (Dianthus species)	Peony (Paeonia species)
Cattail (Typha latifolia)	Peppermint geranium (Pelargonium tomentosum)
Chamomile (Matricaria recutita, Chamaemelum nobile)	Petunia (Petunia hybrida)
Chervil (Anthriscus cerefolium)	Pineapple guava (Feijoa sellowiana)
Chickweed (Stellaria media)	Pineapple sage (Salvia ellegans)
Chicory (Cichorium intybus)	Pinks (Dianthus caryophyllus or D. plumarius)
Chives (Allium schoenoprasum)	Plum blossom (Prunus domestica)
Chrysanthemum (Chrysanthemum morifolium, C. coronarium, Dendranthema grandiflora)	Poppy (Papaver species)
Coriander, Cilantro (Coriandrum sativum)	Primrose (Primula vulgaris)
Cowslip (Primula veris) not American cowslip	Purslane (Portulaca oleracea)
Daisy, English (Bellis perennis) – not American daisy	Radish (Raphanus sativus)
Daisy, oxeye (Chrysanthemum leucanthemum)	Red clover (Trifolium pratense)
Dandelion (Taraxacum officinale)	Redbud (Cercis canadensis, C. siliquastrum)
Day lily (Hemerocallis species)	Rocket (Eruca vesicaria)
Dianthus, clove (Dianthus carophyllus)	Rose (Rosa species)
Dill (Anethum graveolens)	Rose geranium (Pelargonium graveolens)
Elder flower (Sambucus canadensis or S. caerulea)	Rose of Sharon (Hibiscus syriacus)
Fennel (Foeniculum vulgare)	Roselle (Hibiscus sabdarriffa)
Fushia (Fuchsia species)	Rosemary (Rosmarinus officinalis)
Garlic (Tulbaghia violacea, Allium sativum)	Runner bean (Phaseolus coccineus)
Garlic chives (Allium tuberosum)	Safflower (Carthamus tinctorius)
Geranium (Pelargonium species)	Saffron crocus (Crocus sativa) - Not Autumn crocus (Colchicum autumnale), which is poisonous
Gladiolus (Gladiolus species)	Sage (Salvia species)
Hawthorn (Crataegus species)	Salad burnet (Poterium sanguisorba)
Hibiscus (Hibiscus species)	Savory (Satureja hortensis, S. montana)
Hollyhock (Alcea rosea)	Shungiku (Chrysanthemum coronarium)
Honeysuckle (Lonicera japonica)	Snapdragon (Antirrhinum majus)
Hop (Humulus lupulus)	Sorrel (Rumex scutatus, R. acetosa)

Hyssop (Hyssopus officinalis)	Squash blossom (Cucurbita species), especially male zucchini blossoms
Jasmine (Jasminum species)	Sunflower (Helianthus annuus)
Johnny-jump-up (Viola tricolor)	Sweet Cicely (Myrrhis odorata)
Kale (Brassica species)	Sweet woodruff (Galium odoratum)
Lavender (Lavandula species)	Thistle (Cirsium species)
Lemon balm (Melissa officinalis)	Thyme (Thymus species)
Lemon Blossoms (Citrus limon)	Tiger lily (Lilium tigrinum)
Lemon geranium (Pelargonium crispum)	Tulip (Tulipa species)
Lemon verbena (Aloysia triphylla)	Viola (Viola cornuta, V. odorata)
Lilac (Syringa species)	Water lily (Nymphaea odorata)
Linden blossom (Tilea species)	Watercress (Nasturtium officinale)
Lovage (Levisticum officinale)	Wild Oregano (Monarda species)
Magnolia (Magnolia grandiflora, M. denudate)	Yarrow (Achillea millefolium)
Mallow (Malva species)	Yucca (Yucca species)

Gabriel Howearth, cofounder of Seeds of Change, made the following statement: "Give people some fruits and vegetables and they eat for a day. Teach people how to grow fruits and vegetables, and how to save seeds, and those people and their families, eat for generations." Another profound statement that touched me deeply came by way of a blackboard in an organic café. "Food not lawns, Grow don't mow." Imagine that: instead of ornamental trees and green lawns, people grew fruit and nut trees, and all types of vegetables! I believe the world would be a happier and healthier place!

While traveling through the countryside, I often pull over to a field and pick a wild salad. It is very satisfying to me to eat crisp, fresh plants, overflowing with nutrition! I never pick directly from the roadside because of the possibility of pollution from motor vehicles.

Thermal Properties of Foods

Thousands of years ago, both the Chinese and East Indian civilizations classified foods as warming, neutral or cooling to the body. Some of the foods on this list did not exist in ancient China or India and have only been classified in modern times. This information is useful in finding the right foods to balance your body and mind under different weather conditions and varying personal dispositions and physiologies.

Many people tell me that it is too hard to eat living foods during the winter. For the benefit of those people who wish to stay warm on cold days, and those who live in the tropics I have put together the following chart.

Warming	Neutral	Cooling
Basil	Apricot	Amaranth
Burdock root	Beet	Apple
Cabbage	Carrot	Asparagus
Cashew	Corn	Avocado
Collard greens	Fava bean	Broccoli Raab
Cauliflower	Fig	Barley
Cherry	Flax seeds	Blueberry
Chestnut	Grapes	Blue-green algae
Chili pepper (before sweating occurs)	Green beans	Bok choy
Cinnamon	Kohlrabi	Broccoli
Cloves	Lentil	Cantaloupe
Coconut meat	Pineapple	Chlorella
Dill	Potato	Celery
Fennel	Raspberry	Cilantro
Garlic	Shitake mushrooms	Citrus fruits (except kumquat)
Honey	Turnip	Coconut water
Kumquat		Cucumber (very cooling)
Mustard greens		Dulse
Nutmeg		Eggplant
Nuts (pine, etc.)		Grapefruit
Oats		Hijiki
Onion		Jackfruit
Papaya (with seeds)		Kiwi
Parsley		Lemon
Parsnip		Lettuce
Pecans (very warming)		Mango
Quinoa		Melons
Rice		Millet
Rosemary		Mulberry
Rutabaga		Mung bean

Warming		Cooling
Seeds(pumpkin,sunflower,sesame)		Nettles
Tea (black)		Peach
Vinegar		Pear
Walnut		Pepper (sweet)
Wasabi		Peppermint
Watercress		Persimmon
Wild rice		Plum
		Pumpkin
		Radish
		Seaweeds (all)
		Spinach
		Spirulina
		Sprouts
		Star Fruit
	Cooling	Strawberry
	Turnips	Summer squash
	Water chestnut	Sweet potato
	Watermelon (very cooling)	Swiss chard
	Wheat products	Tea (green)
	Yam	Tomato
	Zucchini	Tofu (not recommended)

After reading this chart, you can see why many raw/living foodists who are unaware of the thermal properties of foods might have a difficult time maintaining body temperature in cold climates. It seems that the most commonly eaten raw foods -- almost all fruits and most vegetables -- are cooling. If I am in a cold climate, I will consume warming spices with my meals and save the cooling foods for the warmest time or the most active part of my day. I avoid eating melons in a cold environment because they make it harder for me to stay warm. Similarly, I avoid pecans on hot days because they make me feel even hotter. My hope is that you will become familiar with the thermal properties of some of these foods and use this knowledge to your advantage.

Chapter Four: Biblical References

While you may be familiar with the following stories in the Old Testament, perhaps today you will see them in a way that you haven't in the past. The lost teachings of Jesus, taken from the *Essene Gospel of Peace*, are controversial in some circles, but I am firm believer in their validity.

The Old Testament

Numerous classical commentators, such as Rashi, Maimonides, Nachmanides, and Abraham Ibn Ezra, stated that God's first intention was for people to be vegetarian. In *The Five Books of Moses*, God's **initial** dietary law was strictly nonmeat: "And God said, 'Behold, I have given you every herb yielding seed, which is upon the face of the earth, and every tree, in which is the fruit of a tree yielding seed. To you it shall be for food.'" (*Genesis* 1:29)

The Jews wandered in the desert for 40 years in good health on a diet of manna. When they cried out for flesh, which the Lord reluctantly provided in the form of quails, a great plague broke out and many people died. Some commentators have interpreted this incident as an early warning about the negative health effects of eating meat.

When the Lord promised the Jews a special land in Canaan, He said, "For the Lord, thy God, bringeth thee into a good land, a land of brooks of water, of fountains and depths, springing forth in valleys and hills, a land of wheat and barley, and vines and fig trees and pomegranates; a land of olive trees and honey; a land wherein thou shalt not lack anything in it. And thou shall eat and be satisfied and bless the Lord thy God for the good land which He hath given thee." (Deuteronomy 8:7-10) To me it seems that the ideal diet here was vegetarian too.

The Book of Daniel holds the world's first recorded dietary test. "But Daniel resolved that he would not defile himself with the king's rich food, or with the wine which he drank; therefore he asked the Chief of eunuchs to allow him not to defile himself. And God gave Daniel favor and compassion in the sight of the Chief of eunuchs and the Chief of eunuchs said to Daniel, 'I fear lest my lord the king, who appointed your food, and your drink, should see you were in poorer condition than the youths who are your own age, so you would endanger my head with the King.' Then Daniel said to the steward whom the Chief of the eunuchs had appointed over Daniel, Hanani'ah, Mish'a-el, and Azair-ah; 'Test your servants for ten days; let us be given vegetables to eat and water to drink. Then let our appearance and the appearance of the youths who eat the King's rich food be observed by you, and according to what you see deal with your servants.'

"So he hearkened to them in this matter, and tested them for ten days. At the end of the ten days they were better in appearance and fatter in flesh [more muscular] than all the youths who ate the King's rich food."

Later we find that Daniel was able to interpret the King's dreams when none of the wise men of Babylon were able to do so.

"Then the King gave Daniel high honors and many great gifts, and made him ruler over the whole province of Babylon, and Chief Prefect over all the wise men of Babylon."

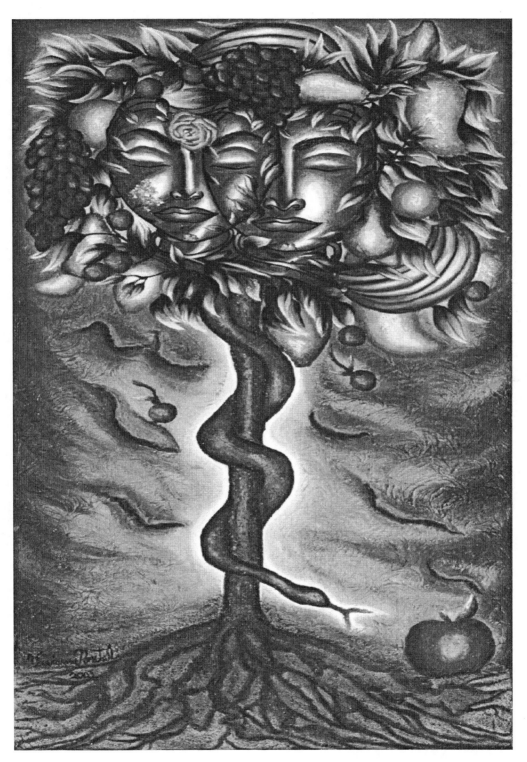

Staff of Life © by Vivianne Nantel, **www.VivianneNantel.com**, **1-866-SOUL-ART**

Jesus: The Lost Teachings

In the 1920's, Edmond Bordeaux Szekely, Ph.D., gained access to the archives of the Vatican and came across some of the teachings attributed to Jesus that are not included in *The New Testament*. His efforts have resulted in the translation and printing of the *Essene Gospel of Peace* into 26 languages. Since then, over one million copies have been sold and the price of this manuscript remains only one dollar. If you have never read it, I highly recommend it!

The contents of *The Essene Gospel of Peace* represent about one third of the complete manuscripts that exist in Aramaic in the secret archives of the Vatican and in old Slavonic in the Royal Archives of the Hapsburgs. The ancient Aramaic texts date from the third century after Christ while the old Slavonic version is a literal translation of the former.

Szekely was a well-known philologist who worked in Sanskrit, Aramaic, Greek and Latin and spoke ten modern languages. Some of his most important translations are texts from the *Dead Sea Scrolls, Essene Gospel of Peace, Zend Avesta,* and pre-Columbian *Codices of Ancient Mexico.*

The following teachings are from the *Essene Gospel of Peace*. On p. 39 Jesus says, "But I say to you: kill neither men, nor beasts, nor yet the food which goes into your mouth. **For if you eat living food, the same will quicken you, but if you kill your food, the dead food will kill you also. For life comes only from life, and from death comes always death** [emphasis mine]. For everything which kills your foods, kills your bodies also."

On p. 40, Jesus gives details about how to make raw Essene bread: "Let the angels of God prepare your bread. Moisten your wheat, that the angel of water may enter it. Then set it in the air, that the angel of air also may embrace it. And leave it from morning to evening beneath the sun, that the angel of sunshine may descend upon it. And the blessing of the three angels will soon make the germ of life to **sprout** in your wheat. Then crush your grain, and make thin wafers, as did your forefathers when they departed out of Egypt, the house of bondage. Put them back again beneath the sun from its appearing, and when it is risen to its highest in the heavens, turn them over on the other side that they be embraced there also by the angel of sunshine, and leave them there until the sun be set. For the angels of water, of air, and of sunshine fed and ripened the wheat in the field, and they, likewise, must prepare also your bread. And the same sun which, with the fire of life, made the wheat to grow and ripen, must cook your bread with the same fire! For the fire of the sun gives life to the wheat, to the bread, and to the body. But the fire of death kills the wheat, the bread, and the body."

Jesus goes on to give nutritional advice on how to stay disease free. "So eat always from the table of God the fruits of the trees [fruits, vegetables, nuts, seeds, beans], the grains and grasses of the field, the milk of beasts, and the honey of bees. For everything beyond these is of Satan, and leads by the way of sins and of diseases unto death. But the foods which you eat from the abundant table of God give strength and youth to your body, and you will never see disease."

The milk was of course, consumed raw, not pasteurized and homogenized. Pasteurization destroys the enzymes needed to digest it and denatures the nutrients. Studies have shown that calves fed pasteurized milk always die. Cows in nature eat raw, unadulterated grass and herbs. Most cows today are fed dried grains that have been sprayed with chemical fertilizers, pesticides and anti-fungal agents and then stored for long periods, sometimes becoming moldy. I do not advocate raw milk today because of the risk of tuberculosis, scrofula and other disease-causing microbes that can be transmitted to humans through consuming raw milk. (Refer to "Food-Borne Illness" in chapter 7 for further information.)

In the *Essene Gospel of Peace*, Jesus also tells people to eat whole food, not processed foods, and speaks of food combining. "Eat, therefore, all your life at the table of our Earthly Mother, and you will never see want. And when you eat at her table, eat all things even as they are found on the table of the Earthly Mother. Cook not, neither mix all things one with another, **lest your bowels become as steaming bogs** [emphasis mine].

"Take heed, therefore, and defile not with all kinds of abominations the temple of your bodies. Be content with two or three sorts of food that you will find always upon the table of our Earthly Mother. And desire not to devour all things which you see around you. For I tell you truly, if you mix together all sorts of food in your body, then the peace in your body will cease, and endless war will rage in you. And it will be blotted out even as homes and kingdoms divided against themselves." He says two or three *types* of food. I believe that means, for example, several types of leafy green vegetables count as one type of food.

Jesus (as well as the ancient yogic teachers) gives advice to eat to two-thirds of the stomach's capacity for optimum health (pg. 42).

"And when you eat, never eat unto fullness. Flee the temptations of Satan, and listen to the voices of God's angels. For Satan and his power tempt you always to eat more and more. But live by the spirit, and resist the desires of the body. And your fasting is always pleasing in the eyes of the angels of God. So give heed to how much you have eaten when your body is sated, and always eat less by a third."

Macrobiotics teaches to eat locally-grown foods and foods that are in season. Over two thousand years ago, these principles were also taught (p. 43). "From the coming of the month of Ijar, eat barley; from the month of Sivan, eat wheat, the most perfect among all seed-bearing herbs. [Jesus was probably speaking of kamut because modern wheat has been hybridized and did not exist two thousand years ago.]... In the month of Elul, gather the grape that the juice may serve you as drink. In the month of Marchesuan, gather the sweet grape, dried and sweetened by the angel of sun (raisins) that your bodies may increase, for the angels of the Lord dwell in them. You should eat figs rich in juice in the months of Ab and Shebat, and what remain, let the angel of sun keep them for you (sun-dried figs); eat them with the meat of almonds in all the months when the trees bear no fruits. And the herbs that come after rain, these eat in the month of Thebet, that your blood may be cleansed of all your sins." To me this sounds like blood-cleansing herbs.

"Eat not unclean foods brought from far countries, but eat always that which your trees bear. For your God knows well what is needful for you, and where and when. And he gives to all peoples of all kingdoms for food that which is best for each. Eat not as the heathen do who stuff themselves in haste, defiling their bodies with all manner of abominations."

Jesus said, "And the flesh of slain beasts in his body will become his own tomb, for I tell you truly, he who kills, kills himself, and who so eats the flesh of slain beasts, eats of the body of death. For in his blood every drop of their blood turns to poison [meat acidifies the blood]; in his breath their breath to stink [Carnivores have very short intestines, so flesh leaves their bodies quickly, but humans have long intestines like herbivores so when we eat flesh it putrefies before it can leave the body and can cause foul breath]; in his bones their bones to chalk [It is now proven that the excess protein in meat can cause osteoporosis] in his bowels, their bowels to decay." (pp. 36 – 37) [Does it not sound like he is talking about colon cancer? The link between colon cancer and red meat has been established by modern science].

Why these teachings have been kept secret in the catacombs of the Vatican for all these years one can only speculate. They make sense to me and I intend to share them, as Jesus may have.

Chapter Five: Noteworthy People
Brigitte Mars

Brigitte Mars is an herbalist and nutritional consultant. She has written several books on herbs as well as the newly released books *Rawsome!*, *Sex, Love and Health* and *Addiction Free Naturally*. Brigitte has contributed the following article titled *Nine Reasons to Go Raw*.

"Many readers have been hearing about raw food diets. For the uninitiated, it might seem like a daunting task. However, for those that make the raw transition, the benefits are many.

Spiritual. Eating raw helps one better tune in to the universal plan, and experience lots of synchronicity. If all our actions are of the highest possible vibration, God can more easily work through us. Living food promotes clarity, and higher consciousness. Emotional stability and happiness increase, as depression is dispelled. A raw food diet helps one feel emotionally healthier, with a sense of well-being and vitality.

Environmental. It requires less land to produce fruits and vegetables than animal products. Animals aren't exploited when one eats a raw vegan diet. Think of all the energy saved from not cooking; less fuel, packaging and pollution! Most of what gets thrown away can be composted back to the earth. In many countries, cooking fires contribute to deforestation.

Flavor. Flavor is vibrant, requiring fewer additives such as salt, oils and sweeteners. There's more nutrients and fiber in raw food. Minerals are not leached out into the cooking water.

Any recipe enjoyed as cooked can be even better raw. An apple by itself is delicious. When baked, it then needs sugar, butter and spices to be tasty.

Beauty. Raw food diets slow down the aging process. You'll feel better, have more energy and need less sleep. Bad breath and body odor go away. One can easily normalize their weight without dieting. Eyes become brighter, voices more clear. Skin and muscle tone improve.

Save Time. Once you get into the flow of raw food preparation, you will spend less time in the kitchen. Many raw fooders ascribe to the "5-5-5 rule:" No more than $5, five minutes or five ingredients to prepare a meal.

However, it is totally possible to make raw food cuisine an art that requires the same amount of time, meditation and preparation as cooked food, yet you never burn anything (including yourself)!

Nutrition. Every national health group (American Cancer Society, American Heart Institute, etc.) suggest we get at least five servings of fruits and vegetables daily. There are more nutrients in the food raw, rather than cooked. Some vitamins lose potency at 130 degrees Fahrenheit. Vegetables are usually steamed at 212 degrees. The fat-soluble vitamins, A, D, E, and K, are destroyed in cooking. High temperatures cause the destruction of Vitamin C and most of the B complex. Vitamin B1 loss from cooking can be from 25 to 45 percent. Loss of Vitamin B2 can be from forty to 48 percent. Cooking disrupts the structures of DNA, and the anticancer compound, indoles. Cooked food loses enzymes, which begin being destroyed at 114 degrees.

Health. *A raw food diet can help one overcome annoying ailments. The raw path has been used to improve the health of those with allergies, arthritis, asthma, high blood pressure, cancer, diabetes, digestive disturbances, diverticulitis, fibromyalgia, heart disease, weakened immunity, menstrual problems, multiple sclerosis, obesity, psoriasis, skin conditions, and hormonal imbalances.*

It is more difficult to camouflage spoiled raw foods than cooked foods*. One is unlikely to get food poisoning from eating fresh fruit or vegetables. No bottled supplement or prepackaged food can compare with the life force of fresh raw food. Raw food requires more chewing, thus providing exercise for the teeth and gums.*

Energy. *Most will experience better work productivity and require less sleep when raw. Memory, ability to concentrate, and reason become sharper Rather than getting fatigued from breaking down hard to digest foods, one will have more energy, be happier, more beautiful and dynamic.*

Economy. *Raw foods cost less, with most raw fooders spending between twenty-five to eighty percent less on food. Better to spend money on good food, rather than doctors, hospitals, medicine, vitamins, and even recreational drugs! Getting sick is expensive. A raw fooder spends lots less in restaurants. It takes less food to satisfy nutritional needs. Raw prevents overeating, however, you get to eat as much as you want, within reason. A big spinach salad, when cooked, becomes a measly portion.*

Easy cleaning. *Imagine never having to clean the oven! Dirty dishes can simply go in the dishwasher after a simple swoosh. No more baked on grease requiring soaking and scrubbing! Grease won't collect on the walls, stovetop and ceiling. You'll find that gentle biodegradable cleaners really work. Never again leave the house and wonder, "Did I leave the stove on?"*

The raw movement is the future. If one can experience a higher state of consciousness, better health, more beauty, eat more delicious food, save time, money and the planet's resources, why not say yes to raw?"

Albert Schweitzer

Albert Schweitzer was a severe diabetic. When he sought the help of the raw food pioneer, Max Gerson, he was ill indeed and taking huge doses of insulin. Gerson took him off his high-protein diet, commenting that since it is the pancreas that has to supply most of the enzymes needed to digest protein and since it is the pancreas which is ailing already in diabetes, why flog a dead horse? Poorly digested proteins only create more than their fair share of toxic wastes. Gerson put Schweitzer on a regimen of fresh raw vegetables and lots of vegetable and fruit juices including apple juice with all its fruit sugar. Ten days later, Gerson judged it safe to reduce his patient's insulin by half. A month later, Schweitzer needed no insulin at all. His diabetes never returned and he remained healthy and very active until his death in 1965 at the age of 92. (This information comes from Leslie and Susannah Kenton, in their book, *Raw Energy*.)

More recent evidence that diabetes yields to raw food treatments comes from Dr. Douglass, Head of the Health Improvement Service at the **Kaiser-**

Permanente Medical Center in Los Angeles. Some of his patients have been able to stop using insulin altogether while others have reduced its use to a minimum. In one of his cases, a brittle juvenile diabetic was weaned off insulin and eventually off oral antidiabetic drugs as well, by a 90 to 100 percent raw diet. Douglass found that some diabetics need to restrict the amount of fresh fruit they eat.

Edgar Cayce

Edgar Cayce, the most famous mystic of the 20th century, would go into a trance-like state during which his wife would ask him questions and he would respond. Out of the 14,879 readings that are recorded and indexed in the library of the Association for Research and Enlightenment in Virginia Beach, 8,968 readings were given for individuals who were concerned about physical welfare. While I cannot find the exact number of people that regained their health due to Mr. Cayce's channeled advice, there were very few individuals who were not helped. Most of the people who regained their health had already tried modern medicine to no avail, and then turned to Cayce. Cayce usually followed a basic diet plan that excluded white sugar, white flour, fried foods and pork. He did recommend lots of fresh fruits, vegetables and salads.

The following are a few examples of Cayce's readings. In Reading #5024-1, a person with gallbladder disease was told: "In the matter of diet, keep away from fried foods. Do increase the amount of raw foods; that is lettuce, celery, carrots, radishes, all of these that are taken as salads." In Reading #1930-1, he was discussing the nervous system. "In the matter of the diet, keep to a great deal of the fruit juices and a great deal of the raw foods taken especially at one meal during the day; whether evening, noon or just which meal depends upon the body. No fried foods at all, ever! The green or fresh vegetables are very well..." In reading #1191-3, he provides advice relative to constipation: "We would, however, be more mindful as to the diet and as the seasons change it will be well that there be more of the vegetables, and at least one or two vegetables or a combination of vegetables taken raw, but fresh."

Each diet prescribed by Cayce was tailored according to the needs of the individual.

Thomas Edison

Thomas Edison, the man credited with the creation of the light bulb, made a very profound statement and one that is relevant to our topic: **"The doctor of the future will give no medicine but will interest his patients in the care of the human frame, in diet, and in the cause and prevention of disease."**

Tony Robbins

One of my favorite success coaches and teachers is Tony Robbins. I was listening to his audiotape series, *Personal Power*, while driving in my camper and heard Tony say the following words, **"If you want to be alive, eat live foods."** He also brings up the point that our bodies are 80 percent water. He says that it only makes sense for us to eat mostly water-rich foods such as fruits, vegetables and sprouts. He explains that proper diet increases one's energy, which is necessary for total success.

Brian Clement

Brian Clement has been an inspiration to my growth process. It was his words long ago that inspired me to take on my current lifestyle. He is the director of the Hippocrates Health Institute.

The Hippocrates Heath Institute is the epicenter of the raw/living food movement. For half a century, the staff at Hippocrates has been helping people to help themselves. Thousands have recovered from catastrophic disease and slowed down the aging process. Hippocrates is best known for changing lives through living food and helping humanity live with more integrity.

Gabriel Cousens

Gabriel Cousens, M.D., Diplomat in Ayurveda, holistic physician, author, lecturer and world peace worker, is the founder and director of The Tree of Life Rejuvenation Center. The Center is an innovative, cross-cultural, live-food, educational, spiritual retreat center and holistic medical "spa" committed to the healing and awakening of consciousness within the individual and the world community. The live-food nutritional protocols, detoxifying sciences and educational programs make this center a true oasis for awakening and healing!

One of the many things that I like about Dr. Cousens' work is that he teaches the principles of Ayurveda for raw/living food eaters. Other teachers of this ancient wisdom that have crossed my path believe that to practice this tradition one must eat some cooked foods (which is completely false).

Richard Schulze

Dr. Schulze is a medical herbalist and former student of the late, great holistic practitioner, Dr. Christopher. Dr. Schulze healed himself of a life-threatening disease and numerous supposed incurable injuries. He has taught many people how to bring about miraculous healings within themselves. He says, "The whole basic principle and foundation of natural healing is not treating a disease. It's creating a lifestyle that is so conducive of health, with your food program, and your cleansing and elimination programs, and your exercise, and your emotional programs, that your body will heal itself."

The following common sense statement seems obvious to me and holds true in every case of illness that I have ever encountered. "It's very simple to get well. You stop doing the things that you did that made you ill in the first place, and you begin new healthy programs."

Both of these quotes come from the "*The Sam Viser Save Your Life Herbal Video Collection.*" I recommend this great work to anyone whose health could use improvement, especially those who have been told that they are incurable.

The Raw Family

Victoria, Igor, Sergei, and Valya Boutenko have been on a raw foods diet since the early 1990's. They have authored many books (see recommended reading section or www.rawfamily.com) and have come up with a few common mistakes that they have noticed among raw-fooders. I have summarized them here.

- Many raw fooders do not eat enough greens.
- Some raw fooders consume too many fats.
- Some raw fooders try to achieve the 100 percent raw lifestyle too fast (the body needs time to adjust).
- Some raw fooders decide that the other necessary components of a healthy lifestyle are no longer necessary after achieving a perfect diet (such as exercising, proper rest, fresh air, sun bathing, etc).
- Some raw fooders overindulge in some foods and neglect a variety of other important foods (fruits, vegetables, etc.) rather than eating a reasonable variety.
- The biggest mistake that some raw-fooders make is listening to the *raw-foods authorities* rather than carefully listening to the very valuable messages that their own bodies communicate to them.

My experience and research leads me to agree with the Boutenkos on these common mistakes.

John Robbins

The most shockingly awakening moment in my early search for the truth on how to achieve optimum health came during a free showing of the movie *Diet for a New America*, by John Robbins. John was the heir to the Baskin Robbins ice-cream empire. Yet he walked away from the family fortune after realizing that the saturated fat, sugar and other components of ice cream were harmful to our bodies.

In the foreword of the *Hippocrates Health Program*, John states; "We have been conditioned to think that only by eating meats, poultry, eggs and dairy products can we be well nourished. Yet research is showing that these are the very foods that contribute so heavily to heart disease, cancer, diabetes, strokes and other degenerative diseases."

Robert O. Young

Dr. Robert Young, Ph.D. in Nutrition, studied microbiology and chemistry at the University level, and has been studying the effects of diet and lifestyle on human ecology for over twelve years. In his book, *Sick And Tired, Reclaim Your Inner Terrain,* he says, "Disease is just an expression of an inverted way of living, eating and thinking." My experience precisely!

He compares a goldfish in a bowl to the human body in saying that if a goldfish's water is not changed and it gets sick, the way to treat the goldfish is to change the dirty water to fresh, clean water. In humans, rather than killing the germs, viruses or treating a disease, change the fluids that our cells are bathed in, "thus symtomatology reverses itself". "Rather than degeneration you will see regeneration." The fluids that he is speaking of are our blood and lymphatic fluids.

Some of his research is groundbreaking. He measures the frequency of foods. Frequency is measured by counting the number of waves of light emitted per second. The more waves of light, the higher the frequency. He found that certain plant foods have very high frequencies. Wheat grass juice, fresh green juices and vegetables are from 70 to as high as 250 megahertz. Hamburgers and chicken have very low frequencies - from 3-5 megahertz. Dr. Young compares the effects of these foods on humans to the computer world saying that computers with higher megahertz think a lot faster. "As we cook food we reduce the frequency of energy of that food, and it becomes dead food. What we want to be eating is live foods." I can say for certain that my brain works a lot faster now on living foods than it did when I ate hamburgers and chicken.

Bradford Angier

A wilderness survival situation is an event that I sincerely hope none of us are ever faced with. However, it is interesting to hear what survival experts have to say about getting the most out of your food. Wilderness survival expert Bradford Angier authored the wilderness survival books, *"How To Stay Alive In The Woods"* (published in 1956) and *"Survival With Style"* (published in 1972). In both of these books Angier explains, "When rations are limited, all foods should be eaten raw or cooked only enough to make it palatable. The longer and hotter a food is cooked, the greater the losses of nutritive values. Even toasting bread diminishes this food's proteins and digestibility."

Rev. George H. Malkmus

After becoming a Christian in 1957, George H. Malkmus completed four years of schooling in preparation for the ministry. During his 30 years of ministry, he pastored churches in New York, North Carolina and Florida. In 1970, he founded the Greater Glens Falls Baptist Church in Glens Falls, New York - a church that grew in six years from nothing to over 600 members. He also founded a Christian school and Bible institute as part of this ministry.

However, at the peak of his ministry, at age 42, he was faced with a life threatening physical problem. He had recently lost his mother to colon cancer, and now he was facing the same diagnosis. His mother, being a registered nurse, accepted the traditional medical treatment of chemotherapy, radiation and surgery with very devastating results. Because of his mother's bad experience with the medical treatments, he sought an alternative. In his search he contacted a friend, Evangelist Lester Roloff, who encouraged him to change his diet rather than accept the traditional medical treatments. Overnight he changed his diet and almost immediately began to get well. Within one year, not only was his cancer gone but so were all of his other physical problems. Since he made the diet and lifestyle change over twenty years ago, he has not experienced any physical problems of any kind - not even a cold, nor taken as much as an aspirin. Now in his seventies, he has more energy than he did as a teenager.

As a result of this experience nearly thirty years ago, he has been studying and researching diet and lifestyle from a Biblical perspective. Based on his research and experience, he and his wife, Rhonda, initiated Hallelujah Acres in 1992 as a Christian health ministry to help alleviate the suffering they were seeing in the lives of so many people. Their goal is to help lead people away from the world's diet and back to God's original diet for humankind. They have brought new hope and health to multitudes with the message, "You do not have to be sick." Rev. Malkmus has taken his ministry to the world with seminars, newsletters, books, tapes, radio, and television appearances, including the 700 Club, TBN, and COPE. Since 1993, Rev. Malkmus has published *Back to the Garden*, a free newsletter that goes out to more than 200,000 households. His books – *Why Christians Get Sick, God's Way to Ultimate Health*, and *You Don't Have to Be Sick! A Christian Health Primer* – have had an incredible impact. Every day, hundreds of people write or call Hallelujah Acres to say how these books have changed their lives.

In the midst of all of his writings and publications, he established a training program for Health Ministers to help spread the Health Message. Over 6000 people from all walks of life (doctors, registered nurses, pastors, lay people, etc.) have completed this training program and now help share the health message with others.

Presently Rev. Malkmus is fulfilling the dream of Hallelujah Acres by proclaiming the message "YOU DON'T HAVE TO BE SICK" to the world as he travels throughout the country delivering his seminar entitled "How to Eliminate Sickness" seminar to churches and other interested groups in person and by television and radio. His books and newsletters are virtually going around the world. You can visit online at http://www.hacres.com.

Yogi Bhajan

Through his teachings on Kundalini Yoga, Yogi Bhajan has helped me evolve into who I am today. Occasionally he spoke on the benefits of living foods. "And I was thinking, I was asking myself earlier what are the four things that I could say on the most important thing that I have learned from my experience to prevent cancer and I have come to the conclusion that at this point I can say there are four most important things. The first one is diet: We have to eat healthy food; we have to eat living foods. I am a vegetarian and I believe as you do that eating meat can't possibly be good for us, but also believe that eating, you know, it is equally important that we concentrate on eating healthy foods, fresh, living foods, foods with lot of water."

Yogi Bhajan lecture, February 26, 1994 (G 662) Espanola, New Mexico.

Byron Tyler

I was fortunate to come across Professor Byron Tyler's quote in the book *Strength from Eating* by Bernarr Macfadden. He states, "All disease is the result of disobedience of nature's laws. It is a crime against nature to eat the food she provides in any other condition than that in which she provides them. Nature does not err. No one can improve upon Nature, yet that's what man attempts to do when he subjects his food to the heat of fire, destroying its vitality and changing its chemical constituents. The product of mother earth, given us for sustenance, are uncooked save by the heat of the sun—the source of all energy. The sun is productive of life. Fire is destructive of life.

"Cooking destroys the life cells in food—the cells which make and sustain life in man. Cook a seed thoroughly and see whether it will sprout when planted. Or graft a dead cutting to a live limb and see whether it will help the growth of the live branch. All live vegetation is capable of either reproducing its own kind or of furnishing life or vitality to other organized living things; take away its life and it can do neither. Life cannot come from death.

"The man who eats cooked food subsists upon the few cells which escape destruction by fire. He is obliged, therefore, to take large quantities of food to secure the required amount of nourishment [emphasis mine]. He is surfeited with material which his system cannot appropriate—dead matter which must be gotten rid of. The system cannot expel this waste material fast enough, and much of it ferments or decays in the stomach or intestines, furnishing food for the germs and bacilli which daily enter the system.

"The raw-food diet prolongs life. Uric acid is now recognized as one of the chief causes of old age. This poison is present to a greater or lesser extent in persons who eat devitalized food, and the accumulation increases with the age of such persons. Another cause of sensibility is the presence of an oversupply of earthy salts or mineral matter in the blood and bones; this is also being produced by eating of emasculated or lifeless food. These foreign substances ossify the bones and obstruct the vital functions, diminishing the vitality more and more.

"By natural dieting these calcareous deposits, uric acid and other poisons, are absorbed or dissolved and eliminated, and their further accumulation prevented. Thus juvenility is retained and 'old age' warded off."

Chapter Six: What to Avoid

In addition to dietary suggestions, crucial lifestyle suggestions are covered in this chapter because healthy eating is only part of the equation in the quest for optimum health.

Nightshades and Arthritis, Oxalic Acid and Kidney Stones

The plant family known as nightshade is of prime concern. These are potatoes (not sweet potatoes, they are OK), eggplants, tomatoes, peppers, tomatillos and tobacco. All contain a substance called solanine, which protects them from being eaten by insects and other living things before they are ripe. Solanine interferes with enzymes in the muscles of humans and can cause us to experience pain. The solanine levels are highest in unripe vegetables but drop as the vegetable ripens. A vine ripened tomato will not cause problems while a tomato picked green and ripened off the vine will. Be sure to buy vine ripened tomatoes and not get tricked by on-the-vine tomatoes. Bell peppers are problematic. Green bell peppers are not ripe; therefore they are high in solanine. Bell peppers turn red when they are ripe and red bell peppers will not cause a problem. This goes for hot peppers also, red is good, green is not. Potatoes are always a problem. When they are harvested they defoliate the above ground portion first. The plant then puts more solanine into the potato to protect itself from the predator. Eggplants should be vine-ripened for the solanine levels to drop.

Solanine should be avoided by everyone but especially those with arthritis and back pain.

Oxalic acid is a substance found in high concentrations in eggs, fish, and certain vegetables (Balch and Balch pg. 483). Diets high in oxalic acid have been linked to the formation of kidney stones in some individuals. The foods that contain oxalic acid should also be avoided by those with joint problems (Balch and Balch pg. 278). Oxalic acid also reduces iron absorption.

The vegetables that I usually avoid which contain oxalic acid are: spinach, beet greens, Swiss chard, sorrel, and rhubarb. When I eat them they leave an unpleasant and somewhat astringent feeling in my mouth. Controversy still exists whether or not oxalic acid is more problematic in raw or cooked foods. I get the same unpleasant feeling when those vegetables are consumed raw or cooked, so I avoid both. There are other foods which contain oxalic acid but they do not cause the unpleasant feeling in my mouth and I believe that they have very small amounts of oxalic acid, so I will not list them here. If you have kidney stones, obtain a complete list of oxalic acid containing foods from *Prescription for Nutritional Healing*, Third Edition. More important than that is avoiding a diet high in animal protein because if you are prone to kidney stones, the consumption of animal protein has been strongly associated with oxalate absorption (Balch and Balch pg. 484).

Each one of us is different. If you are curious as to whether the oxalic acid-containing vegetables are right for you, then I suggest a simple test. On an empty stomach, eat a portion of the vegetable that you wish to test (and only that vegetable, no dressing) and see how it makes you feel.

Genetically Engineered Foods

Very few studies have been conducted to determine whether genetically engineered foods, also known as genetically modified foods (GMO) are harmful to human health. Many scientists believe that genetically engineered foods have been rushed to the marketplace too quickly.

Genetic engineering has triggered food allergies in unsuspecting people. For example, if genes of a particular kind of nut are inserted in a vegetable, a person with an allergy to that nut may react to the altered vegetable. There is no way for us to know if we are getting genetically engineered foods in the United States because it is illegal to label foods as genetically engineered in the USA, though required in many other countries.

Genetic engineering has created new toxins harmful to human health. In 1989, a genetically engineered version of tryptophan, a dietary supplement, produced toxic contaminants. Before being recalled by the Food and Drug Administration (FDA), the mutated tryptophan **killed 37 Americans, permanently disabled 1,500, and 5,000 became ill with a blood disorder** called eosinophila myalgia syndrome.

A British study has found that genetically engineered bacteria lives on in the human gut. Researchers at the University of Newcastle have found that an herbicide-resistant gene from genetically altered soy was found in 3 out of 7 test patients. This development is highly significant because it proves the biotech industry wrong. They have repeatedly stated that DNA from genetically altered foods cannot transfer to human gut bacteria.

Since it is illegal to label foods as genetically engineered in the USA, the only way to be sure that you're getting no GMO foods is to buy organic. Nearly all the nonorganic corn and soybeans in the USA today are GMO. They have been inserting cold water fish genes into tomatoes to provide them with longer shelf life in cold storage. The Frankenstein foods that they are creating should always be avoided if you are concerned about your health. That's why I say, "Just say no to GMO."

Toxins from Cooking

There are an abundance of toxins currently known that are created from cooking. In this section we will only cover one called acrylamide. In 2002 The New York Times reported that cooking most starchy foods actually produces a highly carcinogenic chemical called acrylamide, which is known to cause cancer in laboratory animals.

The Environmental Protection Agency (EPA) currently limits the amount of acrylamide permissible in public drinking water but it does not regulate levels permissible in our food. French fries and potato chips have acrylamide levels several hundred times higher than the EPA allows in drinking water. Yet most consumers have no idea that the process of cooking actually creates health risks.

On June 25, 2002, the World Health Organization (WHO) began a three-day emergency meeting in Geneva to evaluate the recent discovery that certain popular starchy foods, such as potato chips and bread, contain a chemical that can cause cancer (ABC News, 6/25/02). Never before has the agency assembled so many experts so quickly to evaluate food safety. Talking about acrylamide, Jorgen Schlundt, head of WHO's Food Safety Program, told ABC NEWS' John McKenzie: "This is not just another food scare. This is an issue where we find a substance in foods that could cause cancer, and in significant amounts."

Alarms were triggered in April 2002 with the announcement that scientists in Sweden had tested more than 100 food items and discovered that potato and cereal products that were fried, oven-baked and deep-fried may contain high levels of acrylamide, a chemical used to make plastics and dyes that has caused cancer in animals. "It did come as a surprise because it has not been considered as a normal process that you would get acrylamide out of food," said Schlundt. Researchers say it is all about heat. The higher the cooking temperature is, the greater the level of acrylamide. Some researchers blame the acrylamide on the oil present in the starchy foods.

Bread was found to contain 50 micrograms of acrylamide. Cereals, cookies and crackers and potato chips contained 160, 410, and 1,200, respectively. Since the Swedish study, scientists in several other European countries have tested many of these popular foods with similar results.

If you need yet another reason to pass on the potato chips, now you've got it.

Barbecue Blues

Scientific studies have now revealed that barbecued food can be hazardous to your life! The following article entitled, "Studies are revealing the dark side of barbecue" is taken from The Oregonian newspaper, July 13, 2004, published in Portland Oregon, USA.

"Animals develop tumors of the colon, breast and prostate when fed the same chemicals that are created in high temperature barbecuing," says Jim Felton, a senior scientist at Lawrence Livermore National Laboratory in Livermore, California.

Of 40 studies of humans, about 70 percent have correlated increased cancer risk with high consumption of well-done meat cooked at high temperature.

The potential health problems arise from two factors inherent in the barbecuing process: high heat and smoke. Both create chemicals that can cause genetic mutations and unrestricted cell growth that signal cancer.

Barbecue grills get extremely hot, sometimes reaching 600 degrees. When meat is cooked well-done, chemicals known as hetero-cyclic amines or HCAs are formed in the food. HCAs are created when amino acids (the building blocks of proteins) and creatine (a chemical found in muscles) react at high temperatures. In analyzing cooked muscle meats, researchers have found 17 different HCAs that may pose cancer risks.

In 1999, a National Cancer Institute study examined the eating habits of cancer patients. It concluded that eating a daily average of 10 grams of well-done or very-well-done meat cooked at high temperatures increased the risk of colorectal cancer by 85 percent.

In addition to cooking at high temperatures, grills create smoke when fat from meat drips onto hot coals. The burning fat results in hot flare-ups, and smoke curls around the food. The smoke contains benzopyrene, a potent carcinogen in animals, particularly in the gastrointestinal tract.

A 2001 National Cancer Institute study found levels of benzopyrene to be significantly higher in foods cooked well-done on the barbeque, particularly steaks, chicken with skin, and hamburgers.

Lawrence Livermore's Felton says knowledge about health risks of high-temperature cooking began to evolve in 1977, when Japanese scientists showed cooked beef contained "mutagens" – chemicals that change the genetic structure of DNA.

Since then, Felton says, scientists have identified these compounds, learned to synthesize them in labs, and fed them to animals.

It turned out that the chemicals found in cooked beef were as good at causing mutations as any chemical ever found, Felton says "They do cause tumors, some especially early in monkeys."

The April 2004 issue of *Readers Digest* had the following to say about smoked meats: "Smoking was once essential for preserving meat and fish. But hundreds of compounds have so far been identified in smoke, including alcohols, acids, phenols, and several other toxic and possibly even cancer-causing substances...cured meats are high in nitrates – the same trouble-makers in pickling – which combine with amino acids during cooking and digestion to form cancer-causing nitrosamines..."

When you smell that barbecue, remember this article and ask yourself, "is the few minutes of eating pleasure worth the toll this food will take on my body?"

Frying

"Frying food damages otherwise healthy oils. The high temperature makes the oil oxidize so that instead of being good for you, it generates harmful 'free radicals' in the body" (Holford pg. 52). Frying also destroys the essential fats in food, and when consumed, the free radicals produced by frying can damage cells in the body, increasing the risk of cancer and heart disease and possibly **causing premature aging.** Frying foods can destroy Vitamins A and E, which also protect us from these dangerous substances. The damaging effects of frying depend on the oil, the temperature and the length of time. "Scores of unnatural breakdown dimer and polymer products with unknown effects on health are produced by frying and deep-frying" (*Fats That Heal, Fats That Kill*, Udo Erasmus).

Over many years of consuming fried foods, our cells accumulate toxic products for which they have not evolved efficient detoxifying mechanisms. These toxins interfere with our body's life chemistry. Cells degenerate and the damage manifests itself as degenerative diseases.

Microwave Ovens

The microwave oven heats food with the use of electromagnetic radiation. Burton Goldberg's book, *Alternative Medicine, The Definitive Guide* says the following about the use of this kind of radiation for cooking food. "Microwave radiation is not very powerful and it drops off quickly as one moves away from the appliance. Yet, medical science has uncovered disturbing news about the effects of microwave radiation on health...including **eye damage and carcinogenic effects**."

There may be another disturbing side to this modern convenience. Microwaving may cause chemical changes in foods beyond those associated with being exposed to heat. For example, researchers have discovered that **microwaving infant formula for ten minutes alters the structure of its component amino acids, possibly resulting in functional, structural and immunological abnormalities**.

I choose not to build the cells of my body with raw materials (foods) that have been exposed to radiation and suggest that you don't either.

Another important thing to know about microwave ovens is that they leak. Have you ever seen a sign upon entering an establishment that says, "Warning: microwave oven in use"? The old pacemakers were sensitive to the leaking radiation which could have tragic effects on the patient.

If you bought a microwave leak detector from your local hardware store and checked the area in front of your oven while it was in operation, chances are it would not give you a reading. But if you used a TriField Meter (the one that I recommend), you would find that it leaks radiation for several feet and maybe up to ten feet or so. Leakage is allowed to occur because the government has set what they call an acceptable limit on leakage, and poorly engineered leak detectors are not calibrated to show leakage under the 'acceptable' limit. This leakage of radiation penetrates the cells of your body if you are in its path and can damage tissue. For example, many microwave ovens are located above the stove. If the microwave is on and someone is stirring a pot on the stove, the leakage from the microwave can penetrate the lens of the eye, which is particularly sensitive, and may lead to cataracts.

The Owner's Manual that accompanies a new microwave oven states "Precautions to avoid possible exposure to excessive microwave energy". (Notice how they call it energy and not radiation.) They state that it is important that soil or cleaner residue not accumulate on sealing surfaces of the door and that it is important that the door seals are not damaged.

I recommend leaving the room if someone is using a microwave oven and not returning until they are finished cooking.

Electromagnetic Radiation

We (humans) actually have electrical systems inside our bodies. "The nerve impulses that direct motion are essentially a very low voltage electric circuit. Normal nerve impulse transmission occurs at a speed of approximately 136 meters per second, which is fast enough to appear instantaneous to us." (Balch and Balch pg. 276) This electrical system that directs our motion and performs many essential tasks inside our bodies is susceptible to interference from unseen forces that I will explain in this section.

Electric and magnetic fields together are referred to as electromagnetic fields (EMFs). They both generate radiation in the form of waves that become weaker and then disappear as you move away from the source. For example, household appliances generate fields that usually drop off just a few feet away while high-tension transmission lines can generate a field that can travel several hundred feet or more. The fields pass through walls and there is no easy way to block them out. EMFs are found wherever there are electric transmission lines and around the devices plugged into them. They are invisible and silent. Humans are not biologically equipped to consciously detect EMFs; the result of this exposure can adversely affect us. Some people do notice the invisible EMF fields. For example, when exposed to EMFs I need more sleep.

An apartment that I lived in years ago had an electric water heater just two feet from the bed. I almost always shut the water heater off before bed and felt well rested in the morning on seven hours sleep. On the nights that I forgot to shut the water heater off, I had trouble waking up even after nine hours sleep. This went on for several years and I am 100 percent convinced that the EMF field was the cause of the need for more sleep.

Why worry? Spending time in a high EMF field can have dangerous effects on our tissues and cells and has even been shown to cause cancer. Many good books are available on EMFs, such as, *The Great Power-Line Cover-Up* by Paul Brodeur and *Electromagnetic Fields, a Consumer's Guide to the Issues and How to Protect Ourselves* by B. Blake Levitt. I recommend one called *WARNING: The Electricity Around You May Be Hazardous To Your Health* by Ellen Sugarman. The following studies have been summarized from that book.

Dr. Ross Adey, director of the Brain Research Institute at UCLA, and his colleagues found that exposure to extremely low frequency (ELF) EMFs, changed the behavior of monkeys and cats and altered their brain waves. ELF EMFs also changed the level of calcium in the brains of young chickens.

Some people have become so sensitive to EMFs that they have seizures when exposed. This phenomenon is documented in a videotape that I recommend called, *The Current Switch: How to identify and reduce or eliminate electromagnetic pollution in the home.*

What astounds me is the large body of evidence that shows an increased rate of leukemia in humans exposed to EMFs. **The *New England Journal of Medicine* printed a report in 1982 that showed that male utility workers had double the incidence of leukemia in comparison to men in other occupations.**

Several studies have shown a connection between leukemia, lymphoma and cancer of the nervous system in children exposed to EMFs. Dr. Robert

Becker and Dr. Andrew Marino proved conclusively that EMFs cause cancer to proliferate rapidly.

In 1990, **the US Environmental Protection Agency (EPA) tried to warn the public about the cancer risks of EMFs by attempting to label them as a class B1 carcinogen** (the same as cigarettes). They were prevented from doing so by officials at the White House. I believe that this decision was made because the effects of such a label would be enormously expensive for the utility and other industries and would cause an abundance of lawsuits.

But don't panic! You can live a healthy life coexisting with electricity if you follow the few simple guidelines that I will explain. The key to EMF safety is to stay out of high fields. Move your alarm clock further away from the head of your bed; don't use electric blankets, and get a panel screen (flat and thin) monitor for your computer instead of the traditional type. These are just a few of the things you can do to reduce your exposure from very common sources.

In addition to taking these simple steps and most importantly, make a thorough inspection of your own home and workplace to discover whether and where you are being exposed to EMFs. A device called a gaussmeter can measure EMFs. The scale used to read this type of radiation is milligauss (mG). Some experts say that a field of two and a half mG or less is safe. However, it is best to spend most of your time (for example, sleeping, working, and relaxing) in a field as close to zero mG as possible.

I would strongly advise you to buy a gaussmeter or hire an EMF inspector to examine your living and working areas for EMFs. Make sure that these areas and the areas that you spend most of your time in are below two and a half mG. The best and easiest gaussmeter to use that I am aware of is called the TriField meter which measures EMF fields emanating from every direction. Other meters are directional so they must be aimed in every possible direction, every few feet. If you don't do this, a field might be coming from a direction that you do not point the meter towards, so you may mistakenly get a reading of zero when an EMF field is actually present. The TriField meter makes checking for these fields easy and accurate. The TriField is available at www.RawFoodsBible.com.

Cellular Phones

Wireless/cellular/mobile phones emit low levels of radio frequency radiation (RF) in the microwave range and electromagnetic radiation (see preceding section for info on EMFs). Even the mobile phone industry will not claim that their phones are safe. According to Motorola, "It is well known that high levels of RF can produce biological damage through heating effects (this is how your microwave oven is able to cook food). However it is not known whether, or to what extent, or through what mechanism, lower levels of RF might cause adverse health effects as well." My Motorola digital wireless telephone *User's Guide* states, "The available science does not allow us to conclude that mobile phones are absolutely safe."

The same *User's Guide* goes on to list several studies showing that wireless phones can have negative consequences for the user's health. It reads "A few animal studies, however, have suggested that low levels of RF could accelerate the development of cancer in laboratory animals. In one study, mice genetically altered to be predisposed to developing one type of cancer **developed more than twice as many such cancers** when they were exposed to RF energy compared to controls [emphasis added]."

Besides these statements about laboratory animals, the *User's Guide* provides some studies on humans! In a paragraph on brain tumors the guide's author states: "When **tumors** did exist in certain locations, however, they **were more likely to be on the side of the head where the mobile phone was used** [emphasis added]." The guide's author goes on to say that "...**an association was found between mobile phone use and one rare type of glioma, neuroepithellomatous tumors** [emphasis added]."

Many people have explained to me that when using cellular phones they experience uncomfortable feelings on the side of their head that they are holding the phone against. In my experience, when holding a cellular phone close to my ear for more than a minute or so causes me to experience what I describe as borderline painful feelings in my head.

The Nokia 6560 *User Guide* states, in the section entitled Additional Safety Information, "Pacemaker manufacturers recommend that a minimum separation of 6 in. (15.3 cm) be maintained between a wireless phone and a pacemaker to avoid potential interference with the pacemaker." They suggest that users "not carry the phone in a breast pocket" and "hold the device to the ear opposite the pacemaker." For the rest of us, consider this: The human heart beats because of an electrical impulse sent by the sinoatrial node, the pacemaker designed by God. MedicineNet.com gives the following description of the sinoatrial node: "The sinoatrial node (SA node) is one of the major elements in the cardiac conduction system, the system that controls the heart rate. This stunningly designed system generates electrical impulses and conducts them throughout the muscle of the heart, stimulating the heart to contract and pump blood...The electrical signal generated by the SA node moves from cell to cell down through the heart until it reaches the atrioventricular node (AV node)...The AV node serves as a gate that slows the electrical current before the signal is permitted to pass down through to the ventricles. This delay ensures that the atria have a chance to fully contract before the ventricles are stimulated. After passing the AV node, the electrical current travels to the ventricles along special fibers embedded in the walls of the lower part of the heart."

If cellular phones can interfere with mechanical pacemakers, it seems to me that they could also interfere with our sinoatrial node. The symptoms of this interference might appear as fatigue, because overcoming the interference of a cell phone would create the need for the body to exert more energy to ensure proper heart rate. I suggest keeping all cellular and cordless home phones away from your body.

So, how can we make cell-phone use safer? Motorola gives the following recommendations on how to minimize your exposure to RF in the back of their *User's Guide*. "Those persons who spend long periods of time on their hand-held mobile phones could consider holding lengthy conversations on conventional phones and reserving the hand-held models for shorter conversations or for situations when other types of phones are not available." For car owners the author recommends switching to "a mobile phone in which the antenna is located outside the vehicle" (see www.WilsonElectronics.com for this type of antenna).

I prefer and recommend a high-quality hands-free speakerphone that can be placed a few feet away so that one can carry on a conversation as easily as if the person is in the same room. Another device that I use is a specially designed headset. This radiation-free headset has been designed using an air-filled wireless tube that is similar to a doctor's stethoscope. By replacing the wire type headset with a wireless tube, the electromagnetic radiation emitted from your phone can be kept a safe distance away from you instead of directly next to your brain. The device that I am currently using is called the RF (radiation free) headset. Radiation free headsets are available at www.RawFoodsBible.com.

There have been many reports of people living in the same apartment for many years and feeling in excellent health. Then a cellular phone transmitting and receiving antenna was installed on the roof above their apartment and their health declined to the point where they were unable to work. The only option in this case is to move.

On Tuesday, July 19, 2005, CNN TV covered the death of Johnny Cochrane, the famous lawyer from the O.J. Simpson trial. Dr. Keith Black, a well known neurosurgeon from Cedars Sinai Medical Center in Los Angeles has determined that the brain tumor which caused Cochrane's death was strongly connected to his cell phone use.

Following the above recommendations may reduce your risk of negative heath effects but avoidance is the best protection.

Trans Fats, Hydrogenated Fats and Saturated Fats

"Years of dietary abuse, such as in frequently consuming foods cooked in or made with hydrogenated oils, can cause the blood to become somewhat thick and stagnant. Not only is overall circulation slowed down, but artery walls, especially those leading to the brain and heart, become narrower and occasionally clogged with clumps of thick blood and bacteria." (Heinerman pg. 427)

The consumption of hydrogenated oils has been scientifically proven to have deleterious effects on health. The industry uses hydrogenation to add shelf stability for extended periods of time to all sorts of products and to make spreadable margarine. Udo Erasmus Ph.D., author of *Fats That Heal, Fats That Kill*, says, "The process of hydrogenation uses high temperatures, between 248 and 410 degrees Fahrenheit, in the presence of a metal catalyst, usually nickel, but sometimes platinum or copper. Hydrogen gas is added to the oils. This process takes between six and eight hours. The nickel catalyst used is actually 50 percent aluminum and remnants of both metals remain in the products and are eaten by consumers." Some researchers have linked aluminum to Alzheimer's and other diseases.

A study done by E. Hill in 1979 on rats found that hydrogenated vegetable oils elevated serum cholesterol levels while oils in the natural state lowered them. M. B. Katan and R. P. Mensink conducted a study in 1990 to check the effect of trans-fats on high density (HDL) and low density (LDL) cholesterol in healthy humans. Fifty-four young adults were placed on identical three-week diets except that ten percent of the calories in one group were from trans fats and the other group from saturated fats. The trans-fatty acids did more damage to the serum LDL/HDL ratio than did the saturated fat. Not only did LDL increase fourteen milligrams but HDL dropped by seven milligrams in the trans-fat group (in only three weeks)!

The body cannot make use of trans-fatty acids and they block the body's ability to use healthy polyunsaturated oils. It's like a key that fits the body's chemical locks but will not open the door. Margarine, unless stated on the label to be free from trans fat, is made from hydrogenated oils. So I say, "Buyer beware!"

In 1994, the Harvard School of Public Health publicized a study which concluded that trans-fatty acids **double one's risk of heart attack**. This study was aired on all major news programs in America. Also, in 1994 a television ad that had run for years implying that margarine is good for health disappeared. A June 23, 1999 press release from the same Harvard school stated that if unsaturated fats replaced trans fats, each year 30,000 fewer people would die of heart disease (*Fats That Heal, Fats That Kill*, audiocassette).

Until January 1, 2006, hydrogenated fats were mislabeled by a technicality so that the industry could benefit. They were labeled as poly-unsaturated, although they are actually supersaturated. The United States federal government has finally implemented a law that requires food containing trans-fatty acids (hydrogenated oils) to be labeled truthfully.

In Dr. John McDougall's Newsletter, July 2003, he states, "You don't have to be one of these victims of ignorance—trans fats are very easy to avoid. Trans fats are present in small amounts in meat and dairy products. However, the largest doses of these unhealthy fats come to your dinner plate by way of vegetable oils chemically changed by manufacturers to improve shelf life and customer appeal."

"There is a strong association between a high intake of saturated fats mainly from meat and dairy products, and cardiovascular disease. The reverse is true for olive oil" (Holford pg. 51).

Unrefined coconut oil has been shown to be a health guardian rather than a disease promoter! The studies show that unrefined coconut oil contains lauric acid, just as human mother's milk does. This may be the reason that it is added to infant formula. Lauric acid is converted by the human body into monolaurin, which is antiviral. It has been shown that AIDS patients can lower their viral load significantly with the daily ingestion of coconut oil.

Coconut oil also contains caprylic acid which has been successfully used to destroy Candida Albicans (a yeast which can cause yeast infections in humans) in the intestinal tract of humans.

This does not mean that large amounts of unrefined coconut oil are good for you; moderation is the key.

Fats might be the most misunderstood food of modern times. If I could only recommend replacing one type of unhealthy food from your diet, and replacing it with a healthy type, it would surely be fats.

Pharmaceuticals

While pharmaceutical drugs save lives and help many people, they all have side effects and should be avoided if possible. Many people prolong their recovery time from infection unknowingly. You may have the best intentions when you take or give aspirin or other fever-lowering drugs, but by doing so you actually prolong the recovery time and keep yourself or your family sick longer. This is why: When you are sick your body raises its temperature because higher body heat causes the immune system to work more efficiently. For every one degree of temperature rise, the speed at which your immune cells travel is doubled. Immune cells are your white blood cells. The process is called leucotaxis; white blood cells migrate through the blood stream and then through the walls of blood vessels to reach the agent that they must destroy. For example, with a fever of 104 degrees, the immune cells travel 64 times faster than normal to get to the site of infection and destroy bacteria or other problematic agents. Ibuprofen, aspirin and acetaminophen all have the effect of actually suppressing white blood cell activity when white blood cells are desperately needed to help the body overcome infection.

Suppressing a fever goes against what your body wants to do to heal itself. It is a Naturopathic principle that the innate wisdom of the body should not be interfered with in this case. So, unless it is dangerously high, I would not suppress a fever. What is dangerously high? Ask your physician, because the answer differs for every individual, especially for children and the elderly. Before pharmaceuticals were invented people used cold water to lower fevers. Many naturopaths use the cold water method today. If you do have a dangerously high fever, you can ask your physician or naturopath whether this method may be a better option for you.

Another category of pharmaceuticals that may be counterproductive is arthritis medication. Arthritis medication can actually make the illness worse! This is why: Arthritis is aggravated by partially digested food proteins that are leaked through the intestinal tract into the bloodstream. The nonsteroidal anti-inflammatory drugs used to treat arthritis can worsen this problem by making the intestinal walls more permeable, thus allowing even more undigested food particles to leak into the bloodstream. Supplemental food enzymes have been shown to help digest the partially digested food proteins and help sufferers improve their condition. (Food-enzyme supplements are available at any health food store.)

The overuse of antibiotics is a major health problem. The two most important things that I wish to convey to you about antibiotics are:

1) **Antibiotics are routinely given for viral infections and have absolutely no effect on viruses.**
2) **Antibiotics destroy the beneficial bacteria as well as the problematic ones.**

The beneficial bacteria have names like lactobacillus acidophilus, and bifida (just to name two). They are very important and are known for their health benefits. If you must take antibiotics (anti meaning against and biotic meaning life), then you should follow their use with lots of probiotic supplementation (the beneficial bacteria). Either take the beneficial bacterium in the form of dietary supplements from the health food store or make your own yogurt from the directions in the recipe section of this book (most store-bought yogurt has been pasteurized to increase shelf life, thus the beneficial bacterium have been destroyed). Dietary supplements of good bacteria need to either accompany antibiotic use (and continue for a time after) or be taken following antibiotic use.

Some people develop *thick blood* and are prescribed a drug called Warfarin. Warfarin is actually a dangerous rat poison and can lead to internal hemorrhaging in humans! "...Warferin, Coumadin, and related medications are toxic and can produce nasty side effects in the course of time (Heinerman pg. 471). There are numerous plant medicines that can thin the blood while delivering nutrients and promoting health at the same time! See the section in this book entitled Circulation.

Sometimes pharmaceutical drugs can save lives, so they have a very important place in society. However, the overuse and improper use of pharmaceutical drugs worries me.

Vaccinations

Vaccinations do not always perform as promised. In fact, many people believe that they may do more harm than good. In sharing the following information with you I hope to bring to your attention a side of vaccinations that rarely gets talked about on the news, so that you may make an educated decision the next time someone suggests an assault of this type to either you or a loved one.

Vaccines contain both carcinogens and toxic substances. The DPT and hepatitis B vaccine both contain formaldehyde (a major component of embalming fluid), aluminum (a neuro-toxin), and a mercury derivative called thimerosal.

A British medical journal called *Lancet* printed the results of a study which found that people who were vaccinated were three times more likely to develop Crohn's disease and more than twice as likely to develop ulcerative colitis. (N.P. Thompson, Is Measles Vaccination A Risk Factor for Inflammatory Bowel Disease? Lancet (April 29, 1995), p. 1071-1074.

In 1992 a study was released in the *Clinical Infectious Diseases journal* which concluded that every case of polio in the USA since 1980 was caused by the polio vaccine. (Peter M. Strebel, Epidemiology of Poliomyelitis in the United States One Decade After the last Reported Case of Indigenous Wild-Associated Disease, Clinical Infectious Disease, (March 1992) p. 444-449.)

Another 1992 study, printed in the *British Medical Journal* concluded that the Measles, Mumps, and Rubella (MMR) vaccine is associated with an increased risk of arthritis. (C.M. Benjamin, Joint and Limb Symptoms in Children After Immunization With Measles, Mumps, and Rubella Vaccine, British Medical Journal, (April 25, 1992), p.1075-1078)

A study in the Lancet showed correlations between hepatitis B vaccines and central nervous system demyelination. (L. Herroenlen, Central Nervous System Demyelination After Immunization with Recombinant Hepatitis B Vaccine. Lancet, 338 (1991) p. 1174-1175.)

A study in the *Lancet* found that children who received a new measles vaccine died in significantly greater numbers from common childhood diseases than children who did not receive the vaccine. (Michel Garenne, Child Mortality After High-Titre Measles Vaccines: Prospective Study in Senegal, Lancet, (Oct 12, 1991), p 903.)

These studies and more are listed in the book, *Immunization Theory vs. Reality*, by Neil Miller. This book also has many testimonies from people just like you and me. Other good books on this subject are *Immunization the Reality Behind the Myth* by Walene James, *Don't Get Stuck*, the *Case Against Vaccinations and Injections* by Hannah Allen, and *Vaccinations Condemned* by Elben.

Many horrible conditions such as autism, Sudden Infant Death Syndrome, HIV, and influenza, just to name a few, have been linked to vaccinations. Thousands of mothers of children with autism have reported that their child was making clear sustained eye contact before the vaccination(s). Upon getting the vaccination the child screamed horribly and never made eye contact again. Shortly after receiving vaccinations these children were diagnosed as autistic. These mothers are convinced that the vaccination was the cause of the autism and I am too.

The truth is that proper hygiene and better living conditions are responsible for the decline of many childhood illnesses, not vaccinations. If you study the statistics you will see the truth. Childhood diseases have been shown to boost the child's immune system which is more important toward resisting future diseases.

Louis Pastour, the father of the germ theory of disease, said on his death bed: "The disease is nothing, the terrain is everything." What he was finally admitting was that a healthy body (terrain) is the most important factor in avoiding disease. Consider this example: If you took a package of viable seeds and planted half in good soil, watered them and had all the proper conditions for that seed to grow, and took the other half of the seeds and placed them on the pavement with no water, which seeds would grow? Now think of a person with a weakened immune system always blowing his/her nose to remove mucus versus a person with a strong immune system that is mucus-free. There is no fertile soil in the healthy person for the germs to grow; therefore that person can be exposed to germs and not get sick. But the unhealthy person has very fertile soil in which the germs can live and thrive. In my early years I was the unhealthy person with the stuffy nose, always getting sick. Now I am the healthy person who has not been sick in years!

Dozens of books are available that reveal the true dangers of immunization. I suggest getting one and reading it. The time has come for us to boost our immune systems naturally through proper nutrition and lifestyle choices: We can no longer rely on better living through chemistry.

Personal Care Products

Every day we use products that we think are safe, but the truth is that personal care and home care products are not always safe and manufacturers don't always have to tell us so.

In 1938 the Food and Drug Administration (FDA) granted self-regulation to the cosmetic industry. Since then, cosmetics have been sold without government approval of ingredients. The cosmetic industry decided that if less than 50 percent of laboratory animals die while testing a new cosmetic ingredient, that ingredient is considered non-toxic. So to this day, **if 49 percent of laboratory animals die from a cosmetic ingredient, it's labeled as non-toxic**.

Most of the 25,000 chemicals used today have not been tested for long-term toxic effects, not that calling a product non-toxic means anything anyway. Many people in the United States are exposed to over 200 different chemicals each day, many of which are suspected of causing cancer or juggling hormones. Environmental Protection Agency (EPA) tests conclude that ingredients in personal care products and home care products may be wreaking havoc with hormones that control reproduction and development.

In the same manner that trans-dermal patches work, for example, the patch that is placed on the skin to deliver nicotine for people trying to quit smoking, chemicals that come into contact with the skin are absorbed into our bloodstream and brought to our liver for detoxification. These chemicals can build up in the body and can cause ill health.

Alcohol and solvents damage our skin's immune barrier, deplete our skin's moisture, dissolve proteins, encourage bacteria and parasite growth, and accelerate aging. Soaps and detergents strip our skin's precious moisture shield, reduce our body's immune barrier, leave the skin malnourished, and accelerate aging.

The following is a partial list of **ingredients to avoid** in personal and home care products:

Alcohol, Isopropyl (SD-40): A consumer's dictionary of cosmetic ingredients says that it may cause headaches, flushing, dizziness, mental depression, nausea, vomiting, narcosis, and coma. Fatal ingested dose is one ounce or less.

DEA (Diethanolamine), MEA (Monoethanolamine) & TEA (Triethanolamine): Hormone-disrupting chemicals that can form cancer-causing nitrates and nitrosamines. These chemicals are restricted in Europe due to known carcinogenic effects. In the United States they are still used in shampoos, shaving creams, and bubble baths. Dr. Samuel Epstein, Professor of Environmental Health at the University of Illinois, says that repeated skin applications of DEA-based detergents resulted in a major increase in the incidence of liver and kidney cancer. The FDA's John Bailey says that these findings are especially important since "the risk equation changes significantly for children".

DMDM Hydantoin and Urea (Imidazolidinyl): Just two of many preservatives that often release formaldehyde which may cause joint pain, skin reactions, allergies, depression, headaches, chest pain, ear infections, chronic fatigue, dizziness, and loss of sleep. Exposure may also irritate the respiratory system, trigger heart palpitations or asthma, and aggravate coughs and colds. Other possible side-effects include weakening the immune system and cancer.

FD&C Color Pigments: Synthetic colors made from coal tar, containing heavy metals that deposit toxins in the skin causing skin sensitivity and irritation. Absorption of certain colors can cause depletion of oxygen in the body. Animal studies have shown almost all of them to be carcinogenic.

Fragrances: Mostly synthetic ingredients, many are toxic or carcinogenic. Can indicate the presence of up to four thousand separate ingredients. Symptoms reported to the FDA include headaches, dizziness, allergic rashes, skin discoloration, violent coughing and vomiting, and skin irritations. Clinical observation proves fragrances can affect the central nervous system, causing depression, hyperactivity, irritability, inability to cope, and other behavioral changes.

Mineral Oil: Petroleum by-product that coats the skin like plastic, clogging the pores. Interferes with the skin's ability to eliminate toxins, promoting acne and other disorders. Slows down skin function and cell development, resulting in premature aging. Used in many products. (Until recently, baby oil was 100 percent mineral oil.)

Polyethylene Glycol (PEG): Potentially carcinogenic petroleum that can alter and reduce the skin's natural moisture factor. This chemical could increase the appearance of aging and leave you more vulnerable to bacteria.

Propylene Glycol (PG) and Butylene Glycol: The EPA considers PG so toxic that it requires workers to wear protective gloves, clothing, and goggles. The EPA also has specific disposal requirements for PG. Because PG penetrates the skin so quickly, the EPA warns against skin contact to prevent consequences such as brain, liver, and kidney abnormalities. Yet PG is a common ingredient in stick deodorants and a variety of personal care products with no warning label.

Sodium Lauryl Sulfate (SLS) and Sodium Laureth Sulfate (SLES): Animals exposed to SLS experience eye damage, depression, labored breathing, diarrhea, and severe skin irritation. When combined with other chemicals, SLS can be transformed into nitrosamines, a potent class of carcinogens. Your body may retain SLS for up to five days, during which time it may enter and maintain residual levels in the heart, liver, lungs, and the brain. SLS is currently used in 90 percent of personal care products that foam, such as toothpaste, shampoos, bubble bath, and soaps. It is also used in engine degreasers and garage floor cleaners.

Triclosan: A synthetic "antibacterial" ingredient with a chemical structure similar to Agent Orange. The EPA registers it as a pesticide, giving it high scores as a risk to both human health and the environment. It is classified as a chlorophenol, a class of chemicals suspected of causing cancer in humans. Tufts University School of Medicine says that triclosan is capable of forcing the emergence of "super bugs" that it cannot kill. It is currently used in popular antibacterial cleansers, toothpastes, and household products.

Fluoride: Every tube of toothpaste sold in the USA comes with a warning label because it contains fluoride. It is very scary. It reads, "If you accidentally swallow more than used for brushing, seek professional assistance or contact a poison control center immediately." There is no way that one can brush their teeth and not have some of the toothpaste enter the blood stream sublingually.

According to many researchers sodium **fluoride inhibits proper functioning of the thyroid gland and all enzyme systems and damages the immune system**. The following disorders may result from ingesting this toxin: hypothyroid, arthritis in its various forms, lupus, and scleroderma. Ultimately, sodium fluoride increases the risk of cancer and other degenerative conditions.

The Delaney Congressional Investigation Committee, a US government agency that monitors additives and other substances in the food supply, came to the following conclusion: **"Fluoride is mass medication without parallel in the history of medicine."**

Dental fluorosis is an enamel defect caused by an excessive intake of fluorides during the time of enamel formation. While in most countries the first mottled tooth is seen as sign of fluoride poisoning, dental fluorosis is proclaimed to be a mere "harmless cosmetic defect" by Western dental health organizations.

There is now a substantial body of evidence indicating that fluoride induces osteosarcomas (bone cancer) in both animals and humans. Most notably, **a recent national case control study conducted by scientists at Harvard University found a significant relationship between fluoride exposure and osteosarcoma among boys, particularly if exposed to fluoridated water between the ages of 6 and 8** (the mid-childhood growth spurt). **The Harvard study's findings are consistent with the U.S. National Toxicology Program's congressionally-mandated fluoride/cancer study** in rats; the National Cancer Institute's 1990 analysis of osteosarcoma rates among young males in fluoridated versus unfluoridated areas in the U.S., and the New Jersey Department of Health's 1992 analysis of osteosarcoma rates among young males in fluoridated versus unfluoridated areas of Central New Jersey.

I recommend fluoride-free toothpaste. If fluoride has been added to your water supply, as they are doing in many towns and cities, purchase a filter specially designed to remove this toxic mineral. A well maintained reverse osmosis, distillation machine, or an alumina filter is best. Carbon filters do not remove fluoride.

I only use toxic-free personal care products (soaps, hair conditioners, toothpaste, lotions, etc). When using soap, I only apply it to my hands and those places that need cleaning regularly. The only times that I use soaps on other body parts is if they become soiled, because I believe that water alone is enough to rinse most of my body clean and that there are beneficial bacteria that should not be removed.

I encourage you to read the labels on your home and personal care products, and to pay a little bit more for products that will save your health and life savings in years to come.

The personal care companies that I trust to use are Aubrey Organics, Dr. Bronner's soap, and Weleda toothpaste. They are available in most health foods stores. There are other toxic-free products out there; these are just the ones that I use.

Aubrey Organics (www.aubrey-organics.com) offers a free book called *Natural Ingredients Dictionary* that explains more about cosmetic ingredients. Most health food stores will give it to you if you ask for it.

My suggestion to you is to read labels, and if you are uncertain about an ingredient, consider spending a little more time and finding a product that you can be 100 percent sure of.

Artificial Sweeteners

The artificial sweetener, aspartame (Equal, Nutrasweet, Sugar Twin), may provoke a variety of negative health effects: headaches, blurred vision, seizures, numbness, insomnia, memory loss, eye problems, hyperactivity, rashes, ear ringing and slurred speech. Some researchers claim that aspartame causes brain tumors. This chemical has been banned or restricted in Italy, Holland, Austria, Belgium, France and Portugal but is still commonly used in the United States.

H.J. Roberts, M.D., author of *Sweet'ner Dearest*, explains that one of the reasons for the many negative health effects of aspartame is that the digestion of aspartame yields at least 10.9 percent methanol by weight. Methanol is a severe metabolic poison. In one instance 25 people were poisoned to death when they drank wine containing only 5.7 percent methyl alcohol. Dr. Roberts also explains that "senior FDA scientists vigorously protested the licensing of aspartame-containing products for nearly a decade prior to its approval."

"Saccharin (Sweet'N Low, Necta Sweet) has been found to cause bladder cancer in rats and its use has been restricted in Canada" (*Eating Safely in a Toxic World*, Sue Kedgley).

The sugar alcohols: sorbitol, mannitol, tagatose, and xylitol are better choices than the above-mentioned chemicals. There is a possibility of sorbitol and xylitol causing gastrointestinal upset if used in large amounts because the unabsorbed portion can ferment in the gut. If I had a choice between the possibility of an overly active bowel or the side effects from saccharin and aspartame, I would choose the sugar alcohols.

Sucralose (Splenda) is not digestible so it claims to provide no calories. It is made from sugar that has been bonded to chlorine. While I could not find safety concerns about Sucralose in Consumer Reports, I avoid chlorine and filter it out of my drinking water because chlorine can cause damage to the human body.

Stevia is not an artificial sweetener. It is an extract of a South American plant. There are no known problems associated with the use of this plant. It is about 300 times sweeter than sugar and must be used in tiny amounts, for it can cause a bitter taste if overused. Stevia is my sweetener of choice.

Primates (including our own species) are designed to run on carbohydrates and have a natural 'sweet tooth'. Unfortunately, the majority of people consume processed sugar that actually robs the body of precious nutrients. Even worse, we eat artificial sweeteners that can cause ill health, instead of eating the fruits that contain so many essential nutrients.

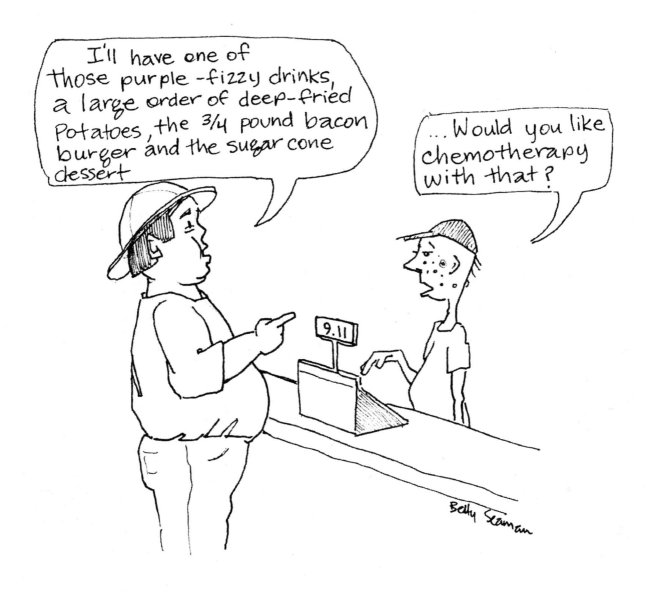

Pesticides, Artificial Colors, and Waxes

Pesticides have a negative effect on our immune system by decreasing T-cells (immune cells) in the blood. You can easily remove a caterpillar from your lettuce and then wash the leaves to remove all traces of the insect. But it is nearly impossible to remove all pesticide residues because they penetrate into the cellular structure of the fruits, grains and vegetables. Washing can remove some residues, but these chemicals are made to penetrate. If they were not, then every time the plant was watered they would come off and need to be reapplied. Peeling cannot remove all residues either because of the penetration factor, and the body needs the valuable fiber and nutrients lost in peeling. Is a peeled apple a whole food the way God intended it to be eaten? I believe that a peeled apple is much better than no apple at all, but not as good as an unpeeled organic one. Many foods have the bulk of the nutrients closest to the skin.

Some foods have been genetically modified to have the pesticide actually growing in the fibers of the plant! No pests will eat it; would you? Corn is notorious for this. The only way to be sure that the food you are eating is free of these chemicals is to buy organic.

Meat is not the answer to avoid pesticides either. Most consumers still don't realize that meat, unless organic, has much larger amounts of pesticides than produce. The grains the animals are fed are very high in these chemicals and are concentrated and stored in the fatty tissue of the animals. If we eat the flesh of these creatures, we are not only ingesting a higher amount of pesticides than in produce but also ingesting other chemicals such as antibiotics, anthelmintics (used to control worms) and growth-promoting hormones-----a chemical cocktail indeed! "Fat-soluble petrochemicals such as PCB'S and dioxin, as well as other toxic elements such as mercury, are transferred to humans predominantly via the fatty portions of fish, dairy, meat, and poultry, and in that order." (Fuhrman pg. 155)

What are the worst foods to eat if we wish to avoid pesticides? Animal products such as beef and chicken are at the top of the list. Far beneath that come strawberries, bell pepper, spinach, cherries, peaches, cantaloupes, celery, apples, apricots, green beans and grapes. At the very bottom of the list, meaning the least sprayed food is avocados. (FDA and EPA data).

One of the most ridiculous facts about pesticides is that the notorious poison DDT, which has been outlawed for use in the USA, is still manufactured in the USA. It is then shipped to Mexico and other countries for use, after which the sprayed food is allowed back into the USA for consumption. This is an example of the power of big business over the people. We lose!

Samuel Epstein, M.D., has done extensive research and written a book called, *"The Politics of Cancer Revisited"*. He explains that Florida oranges have had their skins dyed with 'Citrus Red No. 2' to conceal color variations that would turn the average consumer "off" or toward California oranges, which have a naturally consistent color without dye. He goes on to say that **'Citrus Red No. 2' is carcinogenic** (cancer causing) as are FD&C colors, Blue #1, Green #3, Red #4, Red #40, Yellow #5 & Yellow #6. Citrus skins are not impermeable and the consumer of the dyed fruit is bound to ingest some of the chemical.

Dr. Epstein explains that the waxes used on nonorganic fruits and vegetables can also be problematic because they contain fungicides such as benomyl and sodium orthophenyl, both of which are carcinogenic. Some common fruits and vegetables that might contain these carcinogenic waxes are: apples, cucumbers, squashes, peppers, parsnips, eggplants, rutabagas, sweet potatoes, grapefruits, lemons and oranges.

Senator Don Regal, who was chairman of the Committee on Banking, Housing and Urban Affairs, authored a 343-p. report on Gulf War Syndrome entitled, *The Regal Report*. All of the information therein is available in the public domain. It states that thousands of American service men and women are suffering from memory loss, fatigue, muscle and joint pain, rashes, sores, intestinal and heart problems, and runny noses as a result of service in the Gulf War and that they had probable exposure to low-level chemical warfare agents (nerve agents). In the conclusion of this report is a telling statement: "Non-lethal exposure to pesticides can result in memory loss, and nerve agents are chemically related to pesticides."

In my experience almost everyone can use improved memory. It is necessary to consume the raw materials needed for proper memory function and to avoid lifestyle factors such as stress that can impair memory. Doesn't it also seem logical to avoid chemicals that are known to undermine our memory function and cause disease?

The following two ideas are not considered when so-called "safe" chemical levels are set for humans.

-Exposure to one compound may compromise the body's ability to detoxify another.

-When chemicals and pesticides combine in the body, making new compounds, how can safe chemical levels be set?

We just don't have the answers to these questions and avoidance is the key.

Another factor to consider is that organic produce has been repeatedly shown to be of higher nutritional value than conventionally grown produce. *Consumer Reports on Health,* January 2005 issue states, "...organic produce may possibly pack more vitamin C, calcium, iron, and magnesium as well as various disease-fighting substances called phytonutrients." I will explain why.

Conventional farmers use the cheapest fertilizers which contain only three nutrients: nitrogen, phosphorous, and potassium. The plants need a wide array of nutrients for a healthy defense system against pests. Since they don't receive those nutrients, the farmers are forced to spray poisonous chemicals (pesticides) on the plants to keep the bugs and other pests from destroying their crops.

Organic farmers will fertilize their crops with more expensive fertilizers that contain a wide array of minerals. The organically fertilized plants grow strong defense systems and are not prone to disease like the conventionally grown plants. Pests might eat some of the crop, thus they achieve a smaller harvest, but a superior product is produced. Those are two of the many reasons why it costs more for the farmer to produce organic produce.

My advice to you is not to be penny wise and pound foolish. Organic foods supply superior nutrition and are free from the pesticides and other chemicals that can lead to horrible diseases in humans.

Caffeine

Caffeine can be a useful drug if it is not abused. Those occasions where you find yourself needing to stay awake for a very important reason is a perfect time to use this drug (if you are in good health). It is important not to use it on a daily basis because it can be highly addictive (for many people) and can lead to the following problems.

Caffeine increases the production of stomach acid, alters the metabolism of fat, temporarily raises blood pressure and can cause insulin to be released. It can cause heartburn and stomach upsets and may trigger migraines and benign breast tumors. Heavy caffeine consumers may develop stomach disorders, heart palpitations, anxiety and insomnia. When addicted, caffeine users must have it every day or suffer headaches and fatigue.

The *Taber's Cyclopedic Medical Dictionary*, Edition 17 (pg. 288) says the following about caffeine: "An alkaloid present in coffee, chocolate, tea, many cola drinks, cocoa, and over the counter medicines such as Anacin, Excedrin, No-Doze, and Vivarin...The pharmacological action of caffeine includes central nervous system stimulation; stimulates gastric acid and pepsin secretion; elevates free fatty acids in plasma; acts as a diuretic; increases basal metabolic rate; decreases total sleep time; and may increase blood sugar level....The possibility that caffeine contributes to cardiovascular disease, various cancers and birth defects has been investigated. These studies have not provided definitive answers."

Research at St. Georges Hospital in London has shown that caffeine can cause the muscles around the bladder to contract, resulting in pressure on the bladder. This produces frequent urination in some individuals.

The stimulating effect of caffeine can also lead to sexual dysfunction in men by preventing relaxation in the smooth muscles and nerves of the penis. These nerves need to be relaxed in order to allow blood to flow to the organ. In fact, Viagra works by causing the smooth muscle cells in a man's reproductive tract to relax, just the opposite of caffeine.

Coffee, which is high in caffeine, also contains oxalic acid, even when it is decaffeinated. Oxalic acid binds to minerals in the digestive tract and prevents their absorption, a process which has been linked to facilitating osteopenia and osteoporosis. Oxalic acid has also been linked to the formation of kidney stones.

In the book, *Poison with a capital C*, by Agatha Thrash M.D. and Calvin Thrash M.D., the authors state, "There are at least 100 harmful chemical compounds in coffee including acetaldehyde, acetic acid, ammonia, carbon disulfide, catechol, ethanol, methanol, naphthalene, phenol, and hydrogen sulfide, all combining to make your body an unwitting and perhaps unwilling apothecary...Many people take about 1/10 the lethal dose every day, and even in one cup of coffee lurk substances that seriously alter the body. Women who drink only one cup of coffee per day have almost three times greater risk of getting bladder cancer than abstainers!"

Many people are finding that caffeine has a highly stimulating effect when cooked, but not when eaten raw. One experiment conducted with a decoction of roasted ground cacao beans in boiling water produced an excitement of the nervous system similar to that caused by black coffee. An excited state of circulation was demonstrated in this case by an accelerated pulse. Notably, when the same decoction was made with raw, unroasted cacao beans neither effect was noticeable. I occasionally indulge in raw cacao and find it to be rather satisfying. It never gives me the jitters, but when I have indulged in much smaller amounts of cooked cacao (chocolate), I became jittery.

So why ingest a drug such as caffeine? I find that a healthy diet and a good yoga set provide me with more energy than I usually need and I never have a problem sleeping!

The Crab Syndrome

Many times while gazing into a bucket of crabs, I have noticed that if one tries to climb out, the others will grab it and pull it back down. This makes it unnecessary to put a lid on the bucket. I have also noticed this type of behavior in humans.

When we attempt to change our lifestyle for what we perceive as an improvement, even very loving and well-meaning people behave like crabs in a bucket. I believe that some of these people might feel fearful for us because our action goes against what they have been taught and what television leads them to believe, or they feel threatened in some way. The best advice that I can give on how to deal with these people is to give them more love and not try to jam information down their throats. The more you push, the more (most) people will resist. Let them see the positive changes in you without you pointing them out and only offer information if asked (and even keep that information short). This will keep peace and harmony in the community and make everyone feel good.

Food-Borne Illness

The Center for Disease Control says that food-borne illness strikes 76 million people each year in the United States. The statistics show that food-borne illness is on the increase. These illness rates are 34 percent higher than they were in 1948.

Some foods such as shellfish and the meat and milk of animals can be very dangerous to health if eaten raw. The Food and Drug Administration lists the following bacteria that cause food-borne illnesses.

Campylobacter: Found in raw and undercooked meat such as beef, poultry and shellfish, raw milk and contaminated water.

Clostridium botulinum: Found in vacuum-packed and improperly canned foods. Can be fatal in three to ten days if left untreated.

Clostridium pefringens: Found in the intestinal tracts of animals and humans. Can contaminate food left for extended periods in steam tables or at room temperature via dust particles. Mostly a danger at buffets and picnics where the food is left at 40 - 140 degrees Fahrenheit for longer than three hours.

Escherichia coli: Found in undercooked ground beef, raw milk, contaminated water, and occasionally on unwashed fruits and vegetables (can be washed off fruits and vegetables).

Listeria monocytogenes: Found in beef and poultry, improperly processed ice cream, soft cheese, raw milk, and occasionally unwashed leafy vegetables (can be washed off vegetables).

Salmonella: Has over 2,300 strains; found in undercooked beef, poultry, eggs, seafood, raw milk and dairy products with 350,000 reported cases in humans per year.

Shigella: Known to have over 30 types; found in food and water that has been exposed to fecal contamination.

Staphylococcus aureus: Found in foods that have been handled improperly.

In the August 2004 issue of *Readers Digest*, the information on the following four pathogens was printed in an article entitled, *A Plateful of Trouble*.

Campylobacter: (onset of symptoms: 2 – 5 days post-exposure) Infection can kill if it enters the bloodstream. Can also cause arthritis and Guillain-Barrè syndrome (an autoimmune disorder). Present in more than half of the raw chicken sold in the United States.

Salmonella: (12 – 72 hours post-exposure) Infection can kill if it enters the bloodstream. Can also cause arthritis and Reiter's syndrome (inflammation of the joints and tendons). Usually transmitted by foods tainted with animal feces.

E. coli type 0157:H7 (1 – 8 days post-exposure) Can cause hemolytic uremic syndrome (which can lead to kidney failure, brain damage, strokes, and death). Survivors often have kidney dysfunction, high blood pressure, seizures, blindness or paralysis. Most often traced to contaminated ground beef.

Listeria monocytogenes (9 – 48 hours post-exposure) Can lead to miscarriage, stillbirth. Affected infants at risk for sepsis, meningitis. Avoid unpasteurized milk and juice and soft cheeses like Brie, Feta, and Bleu. Don't let fluid from hot dog packages drip onto other foods or utensils.

Food-borne bacteria are destroyed by heating foods at high temperatures in the case of animal products and by properly washing fruits and vegetables. Many commercial fruit and vegetable washes are available in health food stores. My favorite is grapefruit seed extract (gse), which also can be used as a dietary supplement to kill microorganisms in the stomach and intestinal tract. I knew a woman who led cancer clinic tours in Mexico by van from southern California. She told me that she was constantly getting sick from the bacteria in the Mexican food until she started taking grapefruit seed extract as a prophylactic. From that day on, she never got sick. I also used this powerful medicine while traveling for two and a half months in India. Most of the time I ate peelable fruits and vegetables. When not easily peelable, I would soak them in a mixture of grapefruit seed extract (gse) and water for twenty minutes. When eating in a restaurant, I ingested the tablets as a prophylactic. Every other tourist I spoke with either had travelers' diarrhea or had had it in the past. I only experienced it twice (for a period of only a few hours) when I neglected to take the gse. I then ingested the gse which quickly took care of the problem. I also supplemented my diet with beneficial intestinal bacteria, such as acidophilus. These bacteria colonize a healthy intestinal tract and fight off harmful bacteria. Unfortunately, antibiotics destroy these health-promoting organisms and leave one more susceptible to harmful bacteria. Thus a cycle of getting sick more and more often occurs and may lead to more serious conditions such as systemic candidiasis and chronic fatigue syndrome.

Zoonoses: Diseases of animals that can be transmitted to people. You can catch these diseases in a variety of ways. Some animal diseases are transmitted only through foods. Medical dictionaries and other sources provide the following terminology for the few diseases listed here. Many other diseases exist that are transmitted to people through foods in addition to the ones listed here.

Scrofula: Tuberculosis of the lymph glands in the neck. Formerly, this disease occurred from drinking milk infected with tuberculosis germs; the condition occurs only rarely today.

Tuberculosis, Bovine: The type found in cattle. It can be transmitted to humans through infected milk.

Trichinosis: A parasitic disease affecting muscles and causing nausea, vomiting, dizziness and diarrhea. It is caused by eating infected pork or ham.

Enterococci Faecium: A dangerous bacterium found in chickens, which is resistant to Vancomycin, one of the strongest, last-resort antibiotics. Fortunately, infections with enterorocci are rare compared to salmonella or campylobacter (Holford pg. 41).

Vibrio parahaemolyticus: a seafood-dwelling bacterium that can cause two-day bouts of stomach cramps, vomiting and diarrhea.

Bovine Spongiform Encephalophy: Following is the 1992 New American Medical Dictionary's definition of BSE (Bovine Spongiform Encephalopathy/Mad Cow Disease). BSE is the fatal disease that has affected cows and has been passed on to humans in the United Kingdom. The infectious agent responsible for BSE is called a prion; it latches on to proteins in the brain and changes them. It is now proven to pass from species to species and into man. Creutzfeldt-Jacob

Disease (CJD), the human equivalent of Mad Cow Disease, bears the same genetic markings as those in BSE.

Creutzfeldt-Jakob Disease may have greater public health consequences than the suspected number of confirmed cases might indicate. CJD is not reportable in most states and is often misdiagnosed or omitted from death certificates. Prions are thought to cause CJD. It is extremely difficult to kill these infectious agents. Normal sterilization procedures do not eliminate contamination.

What is it? CJD is a horrendous fatal brain-deteriorating disease for which no treatment or cure exists. Most scientists believe CJD is caused by a prion, which is an abnormal isoform of a host-encoded protein (a protein-based molecule with no RNA or DNA). While there are many forms of CJD, recently, an atypical form, labeled new variant CJD (nvCJD) was discovered which appears to be more closely related to the clinical and pathological correlates of Kuru. (Kuru was discovered in New Guinea and is said to be caused by cannibalism rituals.) nvCJD has been related to BSE or as it is more commonly called, Mad Cow Disease. The incubation period for CJD was thought to be decades; however, recent clinical presentations have shown it could be much less.

Who gets it and how? The consumption of cow flesh is the most common source for the prions to enter the body. CJD affects both men and women worldwide usually between the ages of 50 to 75 years, but can strike at any age. The officially stated mortality rate is one to two deaths per one million of the population per year. However, this figure appears to be an understatement as CJD is often misdiagnosed.

In a study done by Yale University researchers, **13% of Alzheimer patients were found, upon autopsy, to actually have CJD.** A similar study performed at the University of Pittsburgh showed over five percent of Alzheimer's patients were CJD victims.

What are the symptoms of CJD? The initial symptoms are subtle and ambiguous and can include insomnia, depression, confusion, personality and behavioral changes, strange physical sensations, balance disorders and/or memory, coordination and visual problems. Rapid progressive dementia and usually myoclonus (involuntary, irregular jerking movements) develop as CJD progresses. Also, language, sight, muscular weakness, swallowing and coordination problems worsen. The patient may appear startled and become rigid. In the final stage, the patient loses all mental and physical functions. The patient may lapse into a coma and usually dies from an infection like pneumonia; precipitated by the bedridden, unconscious state. The duration of CJD from the onset of symptoms to death is usually one year or less.

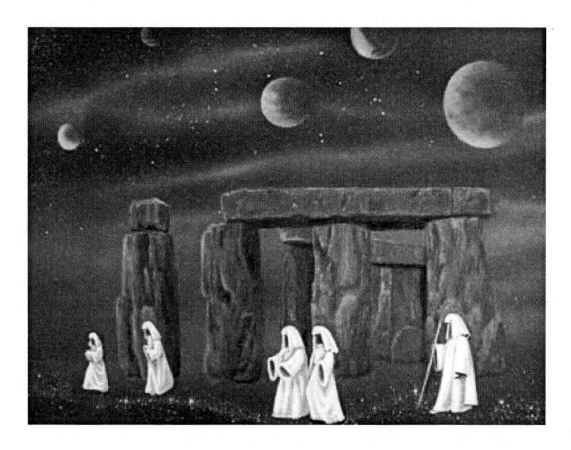

Druids at Stonehenge © by Gwen Ingram, www.eye-dias.com

Rabbit Starvation

Rabbit starvation is particularly well known in the Far North according to Bradford Angier. In his book, *How To Stay Alive In The Woods,* Bradford states, "An exclusive diet of any lean meat, of which rabbit is a practical example, will cause digestive upset and diarrhea. Eating more and more rabbit, as one is impelled to do because of the increasing uneasiness of hunger, will only worsen the condition. The diarrhea and the general discomfort will not be relieved unless fat is added to the diet. Death will follow, otherwise, within a few days. One would probably be better off on just water than on rabbit and water."

The fact that a diet made up of exclusively lean meat can kill humans may be one of the reasons that high protein/low carbohydrate diets are laden with fat and also why modern meat production is producing extremely fat-laden meat.

Chapter 7:
Recommendations for Healthy Living

(Some of the topics in this chapter are not related to what you eat but are crucial in the quest for optimum health.)

Acid-Alkaline Balancing

Maintaining the human body's pH is extremely important. The pH of the human bloodstream is approximately 7.4. If the pH of the bloodstream increases or decreases by just a small amount, we will die. Lucky for us we store calcium, magnesium and other minerals in our bones that are used to buffer the acidity of our bloodstream. **Our diet should be composed of about 80% alkaline-forming foods and 20% acid-forming foods. The standard American diet (SAD) is reversed at about 80% acid-forming and 20% alkaline-forming.** The acid condition in the body that the SAD diet causes pulls calcium out of our bones to buffer the acidity of the bloodstream and can lead to osteopenia or osteoporosis. As has been proven frequently, the answer is not more calcium, but rather proper diet.

One thing that determines if a food is acid- or alkaline-forming is the mineral content or ash that is left over after the food has been digested. The following common minerals are alkaline-forming to the tissues in our body: calcium, iron, magnesium, potassium and sodium. Some acid-forming minerals are chlorine, phosphorus and sulfur. Another factor that determines how a food affects our pH is the protein level. Amino acids (building blocks of protein), when eaten to excess, cause our urine to become more acidic. The body then pulls alkaline minerals out of the bloodstream to buffer the pH of the urine. This process acidifies the body by stealing alkaline minerals such as calcium and magnesium. Another factor that must be considered is that other elements of foods besides minerals and protein levels, such as acids and sugars, can have an acidifying effect on the tissues of our bodies. Citrus foods and sugar may be acid-forming to us even though up until now the scientific community has classified them as alkaline forming.

Whether the food is acidic or alkaline in the stomach has little to do with whether it has an acidifying or alkalinizing effect on the tissues of the body. Milk is alkaline in the stomach but acidifying to the tissues after digestion because it contains a high amount of protein (amino acids). In general, all animal meat, milk and eggs, common grains (wheat, rye, barley), and sugar are acid-forming, and almost all fresh, raw fruits and vegetables are alkaline-forming. I have included a chart for easy viewing. This chart is not 100% accurate, because the mineral content of different soils varies causing the mineral content of the food grown in it to vary as well.

Recent research has shown that negative emotions have an acidifying effect on our tissues while positive emotions have an alkalizing effect on us. So it seems to be just as important to choose love over fear as it is to choose our foods wisely.

Acid-forming Foods	Alkaline-forming Foods
Alcoholic beverages	Avocado
Beans (most)	Carrots
Buckwheat	Cinnamon
Chickpeas	Coconut (young fresh meat)
Chocolate	Currants
Coconut (dried meat)	Dates
Coffee	Dulse
Condiments (catsup and mustard)	Figs
Cranberries	Fruit (most)
Dried sulfur-preserved fruits (most)	Ginger
Eggs	Honey (raw)
Fish and Shellfish (all)	Horseradish
Flour products (bread and pasta)	Lima beans
Grains (most, unsprouted)	Maple syrup
Legumes	Millet
Lentils	Miso
Meat (chicken, fish...)	Molasses
Milk products (ice cream, cheese, etc.)	Mushrooms
Nuts (peanuts, cashews, chestnuts)	Nori
Oats	Onions
Olives (olive oil)	Quinoa
Plums (prunes)	Raisins
Rice	Salt
Sauerkraut	Sea vegetables
Seeds (most)	Sprouts
Soda	Strawberries
Sugar	Sweet potatoes
Tea (black)	Umeboshi plums
Vinegar	Vegetables (almost all)

Our diet should be composed of about 80% alkaline-forming foods and 20% acid-forming foods.

Cleansing Reactions / The Healing Process

After years of being on the SAD (Standard American Diet), most people need to gradually switch over to a healthy diet, and more importantly, cleanse the intestinal tract and get it functioning properly first. When your intestinal tract is functioning optimally, you will have an unforced bowel movement after every meal (just like a baby).

Dr. Richard Anderson's book, *Cleanse & Purify Thyself (book one),* explains the negative side of a quick dietary transition without opening the eliminative channels first. "The problem with going on a raw-food diet without cleansing is this: When the average person goes on raw foods, even for a few days, the body begins to cleanse. What's wrong with that? Well, it brings up cleansing reactions. The average person is full of toxic waste that a completely raw-food diet, without complete intestinal cleansing, could stir up more problems than most people want to handle. Fruits are the most cleansing of all. Vegetables do not cleanse nearly as rapidly. It is ironic that because of cleansing reactions, it sometimes appears that eating fresh raw food makes a person sick, while eating cooked or junk foods makes a person feel temporarily better. All that has really happened in this scenario, however, is that the eating of junk foods has stopped the cleansing process."

"Cleansing reactions on a raw-food diet, without cleansing the digestive tract first, can be so severe for the average person, that a lack of energy, a 'spacey' feeling, eruptions of the skin, and overloads on the kidneys, liver and other organs can be weakening to the point of ineffectiveness."

Dr. George Malkmus explains in his videotape, *How To Eliminate Sickness,* that when we stop eating the "worldly garbage" (chemical-laced, over-processed, cooked foods and so forth), the body has a chance to flush the built-up toxins out of the tissues for disposal. He jokingly claims that the body says, "Whoopee! It's time to clean house!"

I do not recommend a pregnant woman dramatically change her diet to raw foods because the toxins released from storage in her body could possibly harm the fetus or shock the system in such a way as to trigger a miscarriage.

My advice to you: **transition slowly**. If you feel cleansing reactions at inappropriate times, back off a bit by eating foods like steamed vegetables and brown rice. Don't assume that all problems or symptoms are cleansing reactions. If they are severe or persist, see your allopathic doctor (regardless of what anyone says) because they have been thoroughly trained in the art of diagnosis.

Remember: cleansing reactions should only be temporary. After they run their course, you might feel better than you have ever felt in your life!

Brian Clement has come up with guidelines for understanding the processes taking place inside your body during your detoxification. "Actually, 60 percent of accumulated wastes will be released in the first seven days of your program [the Hippocrates Health Program], but complete healing and restoration of the body takes a number of years and breaks down into stages of 7-year increments. It will take the first seven years to completely rebuild the body in the following phases.

1 day-1½ years....Digestive cleansing-major fat deposits and calcifications removed.

1½-2 years...........Deep tissue cleansing and joint cleansing.

2-5 years................Bone structure, cartilage, and further joint cleansing.

5½-6¼ years.........Organ re-positioning and renewal.

6¼-7 years...........Brain tissue and neurological cleansing.

Cleansing reactions may ensue as layer after layer is stripped away. But you will feel better and better as time passes. Due to the body's cellular intelligence, every part is affected by the whole. And, when one part is renewed, this leads to greater and greater integrity and harmony within the whole being." (Clement, pg. 54)

My digestive cleansing process took approximately one year. In that year, every time I had a bowel movement it felt as if my feces were coated with sand. This was the accumulation of 30 years of eating the SAD diet. During that 30 years sometimes I consumed cold pizza leftovers for breakfast, fast food chicken sandwiches at 2:00am, and chunks of cheese the size of ping-pong balls. I almost always consumed a full meal late at night before bed. The result of that diet was the debris that took a year to come out from my intestine. Now, instead of a spare tire, I have a washboard stomach!

The Liver / Gallbladder Flush

The liver filters all materials that enter our bloodstream. Those materials include airborne chemicals that we breathe, chemicals that are absorbed through our skin, and chemicals that we unknowingly or knowingly, eat or drink. Did you know that most commercial soaps, shampoos and lotions contain chemicals that penetrate the skin and are sent to the liver for detoxification? These chemicals can overburden the liver. I recommend using soaps and shampoos that are free of artificial colors and fragrances. In other words, if there is any word on the ingredient list that you are unfamiliar with, you should take the time to find out what it is. These products are available at almost any health food store in the United States. (Refer to the *Personal Care Products* section.)

Dr. Richard Schulze has put together an amazing videotape set called, *The Sam Viser Save Your Life Herbal Video Collection*. In section 40 of the collection, he explains how to flush the liver and gallbladder. Dr. Schulze recommends that adults do this cleanse four times per year, once per season. It is very easy to do. You just drink a simple and very inexpensive mixture on an empty stomach upon awakening for breakfast and follow it with 2 cups of herbal tea. Consume nothing else until lunch. Do this every day for one week. Lunches and dinners that week should be simple raw meals or for a more powerful flush, fast on water or live juices after the concoction the middle three days. That's it!

These are Dr. Schulze's directions for making the gallbladder cleanse: For spring and summer cleansing, mix in a blender 8oz of distilled water, 8oz of fresh-squeezed citrus juice, orange, tangerine, lemon, grapefruit, or lime, or a mixture of these, one clove of garlic, a one-inch piece of ginger and one tablespoon of cold-pressed, extra-virgin oil olive oil. For the fall and winter cleanse the mixture is the same except that you should use fresh pressed apple and grape juice instead of citrus. To complete the cleanse, after drinking the mixture, wait 15-30 minutes and then drink 2 cups (16oz) of either an herbal detox tea or digestive tea. Once the liver has flushed itself out, the tea pushes it all through. These teas are available from your local health food store. I recommend the Yogi Tea brand. If you would like to increase the intensity of the detox, after a few days on the cleanse, double up on the garlic and olive oil. If you get nauseous, increase the ginger and drink your tea sooner.

Dr. Schultze says that if the citrus is organic, it's a good idea to throw a piece of the peel into the blender too, because citrus peels have essential oils that stimulate your liver and help it produce more bile. The citrus even helps clean the kidneys and bladder. Garlic is a broad-spectrum antibiotic, antiviral, gets rid of [some] parasites, and disinfects the whole system. Ginger stimulates circulation and helps to prevent nausea.

I often see people with dark circles under their eyes, which could mean that the liver is overworked. It makes perfect sense to me to keep this organ functioning properly for optimum health, and this cleanse can help do just that!

Pure Water

Just as important as obtaining pure water is the material of the container in which you store your water. I drink my water out of glass bottles. Have you ever noticed when drinking water out of plastic bottles that you can sometimes taste plastic? That is because the plastic has leached into the water. Many people use Lexan Polycarbonate Nalgene bottles because they are clear, lightweight, and sturdy. Polycarbonate plastic bottles are standard equipment for millions of hikers and babies. They are usually labeled #7 on the bottom; Nalgene is the best-known producer. Since polycarbonate bottles don't impart a taste to fluids, many users assume they are safer than bottles made out of other kinds of plastic. But now an accidental discovery has cast doubt on their safety: www.sierraclub.org/sierra/200311/lol5.asp. The amount of leaching increases as the plastic ages and is degraded by use. A separate study published in *Environmental Health Perspectives* confirmed this finding, and also detected leaching from new polycarbonate plastic.

Many studies have shown that the plastic residues leached from water bottles can wreak havoc in our bodies. If you must drink out of a plastic water bottle, be sure to keep it out of the sun as the sunlight has been shown to increase the amount of chemicals leached. For detailed information on toxic free choices for storing water on a large scale, I suggest the book, *Water Storage*, by Art Ludwig: www.oasisdesign.net/water/storage. If you are unable to carry a glass water container, then stainless steel containers seem to be a safe choice.

The chemicals commonly added to water in the USA should always be avoided. (For the reasons to avoid fluoridated water see the *Person Care Products* section.) Chlorine, although effective in killing some of the disease-causing bacteria, provides the drinker with byproducts that are known carcinogens. Chlorinated drinking water causes at least 4,200 cases of bladder cancer and 6,500 cases of rectal cancer a year in the United States (Ludwig, pg 10).

Tap water in the United States usually contains toxic and inorganic minerals that the body cannot use such as; copper, iron, lead, and other naturally occurring heavy metals. Chemicals that leach into our water may include; asbestos, cyanides, fertilizers, herbicides, industrial chemicals, and pesticides. Biological contaminants that can show up in our water supply include bacteria, parasites, and viruses. Pharmaceutical drugs have been showing up in tap water recently.

As if those contaminants weren't enough, most of the ground water in the United States has been polluted with a highly carcinogenic and immune system depressing chemical called MTBE. (Balch and Balch p. 37) MTBE, an additive in gasoline, cannot be removed from drinking water with either reverse osmosis or carbon block water filters. The only way that I am aware of easily removing 100% MTBE from your drinking water is through distillation.

Distillers are available with glass or stainless steel holding tanks to store the water. To add minerals back to the water that distilling has removed, squeeze a few drops of lemon or lime into the water or add a tiny pinch of unprocessed sea salt.

Because not everyone has the ability to own a distiller or a reverse osmosis filter, I suggest doing the best that you can. Reverse osmosis filters are the second best type and solid carbon block filters are the third. Experts agree that the most important thing is that we do not drink tap water. Always use cold water for the purposes of rinsing foods if you are not using filtered water. Hot tap water can leach higher amounts of lead or other metals from plumbing or the hot water tank. If you're concerned about elevated lead levels in your water, run the tap until the water becomes colder before using it. In my opinion, the best resource for deciding what type of water filter suits you best is the book, *Water the Ultimate Cure* by Steven Meyerowitz. Steven also explains the harmful effects of dehydration.

For those who live in unpolluted wilderness areas outside the USA, I suggest using spring water that flows from deep within the earth.

Dehydration can cause numerous symptoms which include headaches, muscle aches, loss of energy, and eventually diseases which can be life threatening. The book, *Your Body's Many Cries for Water* by F. Batmanghelidj M.D., has more detailed information on the effects of dehydration. Every time you consume a caffeinated beverage you increase your body's need for water because caffeine acts as a diuretic. Most experts suggest that we consume at least eight, 8 ounce glasses of pure water every day. **We need approximately ½ our body's weight in ounces of pure water every day.**

Oxygen / Deep Breathing

Everyone knows that we can live without food for quite a while but without oxygen we lose consciousness and die very quickly. What most people don't know is that we can control the amount of oxygen that we bring to our tissues, and that the amount has a potent effect on our health.

Most people breathe much more shallowly than is optimal. Our brain is between 1 and 3 percent of our body weight but requires about 20 percent of our oxygen intake. The brain needs oxygen to perform all its tasks, and if there is an insufficient supply, our thinking process will be impaired. However, slow, deep breathing that fills our lungs with this life-giving substance allows our bloodstream to absorb more oxygen and to transport it to our brain for optimal brain function.

Experts in the field say that our bodies require oxygen to produce as much as 95% of the energy that we need. If adequate amounts of oxygen are not available, it may result in a lactic acid buildup. Scientists have found that injecting calm people with lactic acid can cause them to experience panic attacks. So it seems that lactic acid buildup from inadequate oxygen (due to shallow breathing and/or poor circulation and from spending time in low oxygen environments such as sealed rooms) can be a primary cause of anxiety. Antidepressant drugs actually make the problem worse because these pharmaceuticals may deplete oxygen levels even further. They also cause people to become more dependent on the drugs. Thus a vicious cycle is created. Chronic anxiety and depression seems not to come from the mind but from the cells.

For vibrant health, the bloodstream must be able to carry optimum amounts of oxygen. Research has shown that a diet containing saturated fats from animal products (including cow's milk and fish) and hydrogenated or cooked vegetable fats lessens the oxygen-carrying capacity of the blood, resulting in less oxygen to the brain, muscles, organs and so forth. Research has also shown that a diet high in dark green, leafy vegetables increases the oxygen-carrying capacity of the blood, resulting in more oxygen delivered to vital organs.

Deep breathing increases the amount of oxygen delivered to the lungs for absorption into the bloodstream and ultimately into the tissues of the body. Most people take very shallow breaths and do not use the full capacity of their lungs. I recommend full inhales and exhales whenever possible.

Breathing through the mouth is like drinking from a dirty puddle without filtering the water first. The reason for this is that your lungs need warm moist air. When we breathe through the nostrils the air is warmed, moistened and filtered through the sinuses. The sinuses produce mucus to catch airborne debris. If we breathe through the mouth we bypass this wondrous filter. That is why it is important to breathe through your nostrils.

It has been said that our lymphatic system is the body's sewer system. It cleans up most of the waste products of cellular metabolism. The body contains about four times as much lymphatic fluid as blood. If our lymphatic system were to shut down for only 24 hours, we would die. The lymphatic system does not have a pump like the bloodstream has. The only way that the lymph fluid gets pumped through the tissues of the body is by muscular movement such as exercise and/or deep breathing, which both move the lymphatic fluid extremely well.

So breathe deeply and remember that air is free!

Circulation

Poor blood circulation leads to many degenerative trends, including rapid aging. I will explain how this happens and how to avoid such a fate in this section.

Many people are aware that if an artery leading to the heart gets clogged we experience a heart attack, or if an artery leading to the brain gets clogged we experience a stroke. Very few people, however, are aware of the fact that before this happens numerous tiny capillaries become clogged, and this leads to aging. These tiny capillaries lead to every organ and skin cell in your body. Some are so small that the blood cells may only pass through in single file. It only takes a tiny bit of plaque or a blood clot to clog these tiny capillaries. If the cells depending on the oxygen supply from the capillary that has been clogged are suffocated for long enough, they die. Some people theorize that we might feel a twinge of discomfort or pain in the spot where this happens. Our eyes have tiny capillaries through which the blood brings oxygen and nutrients in a single file line of blood cells. When these tiny capillaries get clogged, our vision becomes worse. When they lead to the brain, our memory or other cognitive functions become poorer. When it happens in our ears, hearing can worsen. When it happens to the spine, the back may go out, and so on.

What we want to aim for is optimal circulation, to keep all the cells in our body alive and well nourished. The living-foods lifestyle, provided that fat consumption is not in excess, does just that! There are many foods that can help improve circulation. Fresh pineapple, ginger root, fresh rosemary, daikon radish, cayenne pepper, garlic, and the dark green leafy vegetables (high in chlorophyll) are just a few of the commonly available foods that can stimulate circulation.

Some medical doctors recommend a baby aspirin a day to improve circulation, but aspirin suppresses white blood cell activity, weakening your immune system, and can be harmful to your liver.

If you want to take pills to improve your circulation, the previously mentioned herbs are available in most health food stores in pill form. Other supplements that can improve circulation are coenzyme Q10, vitamin E (d-alpha-tocopherol, not dl-alpha-tocopherol), ginkgo biloba extract (do not ingest leaf powder, use only extract), bromelain, hawthorne berry, gotu kola (herb), and chlorophyll. Suppository chelation with EDTA has also been shown to improve circulation. See www.rawfoodsbible.com for more on EDTA suppository chelation.

What we want to avoid are all cooked fats (vegetable as well as animal) and all the chemical additives that are so common in processed foods. These are notorious for clogging circulation. The only oils that I use are cold-pressed oils, and I use them in reasonable amounts.

A common naturopathic practice for cleaning out the capillaries is a form of hydrotherapy. It simply consists of alternate hot and cold baths or showers or a combination of the two. Start out very gradually at first, say 30 seconds hot and 30 seconds cold, and repeat this four times. After you get used to it, make the cold a little colder and the hot a little hotter, and spend 60 seconds in each. Repeat this six times. Always finish with warm to hot water after this form of hydrotherapy. I often travel to hot springs that are alongside cold rivers and enjoy this form of hydrotherapy.

If the cold water is cold enough and the hot water is hot enough, you will experience a feeling of *pins and needles* when soaking in the hot after the cold. This occurs because the cold water causes the blood to migrate to the inner parts of the body to maintain body temperature and the hot water causes the blood to rush to the surface of the skin in an attempt to cool the body. This causes the capillaries to open widely and then constrict with each change of temperature. The result is that plaque may eventually loosen and/or come off. Finishing with warm to hot water will keep the capillaries open for several minutes to allow the circulatory system to filter out the plaques rather than having them deposit in other capillaries. I suggest doing this every day if you have circulation problems and once per week for healthy maintenance. You should avoid hydrotherapy, except under medical supervision, if you have a heart condition or abnormal blood pressure.

Our blood needs adequate amounts of water to function properly. A dehydrated condition will not allow optimal oxygen and nutrient delivery to the cells of our body. Therefore, proper hydration is crucial for optimal circulation.

Indoor Air Pollution

Fifty million people in the United States suffer from respiratory illness. Asthma is at an all time high. Knowledge is the key to preventing and reversing respiratory illnesses. As you read on, you will understand that there are some very simple and inexpensive ways to take action.

My favorite book on the topic of indoor air pollution is, *How to Grow Fresh Air* by Dr. B. C. Wolverton. Dr. Wolverton states, "During smog alerts people are generally advised to stay indoors. Yet modern scientific research indicates that the indoor environment may be as much as ten times more polluted than the outdoor environment." **The U.S. Environmental Protection Agency (EPA) has ranked indoor air pollution as one of the top five threats to public health.** The U.S. Environmental Protection Agency sets no guidelines for volatile organic compounds in non-industrial settings

The EPA estimates that indoor air pollution from chemicals such as those released by paint are responsible for more than 11,000 deaths from cancer, kidney failure, and respiratory collapse each year. That freshly painted smell that you get when you freshen a room with conventional solvent based (latex or oil) paint comes from volatile organic chemicals (VOCs). VOCs make up as much as 60% of the ingredients in paint and include formaldehyde, benzene, and acetone. These chemicals can cause a wide range of health problems including allergies, headaches, dizziness, asthma, chronic fatigue, liver problems and even cancer. Yet the U.S. Environmental Protection Agency sets no guidelines for VOCs in non-industrial settings.

There are some alternatives to conventional paint. Some companies have come out with low VOC lines of paint as well as sealers to stop existing paint from off-gassing. These paint lines are a significant improvement, but they are still based on manufactured chemicals and may not be an adequate solution for many people. An even healthier and perhaps also more beautiful option is to use natural paints. You can easily make these paints yourself, or you can buy them ready-made, just like any other paint.

To buy natural paints contact: The Old Fashioned Milk Paint Co. Groton, MA, www.MilkPaint.com or BioShield, Santa Fe, NM, www.BioShield.com.

Other common household sources of chemical vapors, (VOCs), include carpeting, ceiling tiles, chlorinated tap water, cleaning products, cosmetics, draperies, fabrics, floor coverings, gas stoves, grocery bags, permanent-press clothing, plywood, particleboard, stains and varnishes, tobacco smoke, upholstery, wallpaper and many more.

Some of the chemical vapors that off-gas from these items and are harmful to humans include ammonia, benzene, chloroform, formaldehyde (embalming fluid), trichloroethylene, phthalates, and xylene/toluene. These vapors can cause Sick Building Syndrome. The symptoms of Sick Building Syndrome include allergies, asthma, eye, nose and throat irritations, fatigue, headache, nervous system disorders, respiratory congestion, sinus congestion and many more.

One way to reduce the inhalation of these chemicals is to increase ventilation by opening windows and doors. Another way is to become knowledgeable about the sources and avoid them. However, it is not always possible or cost-effective to achieve suitable ventilation (for example, during winter in a very cold climate). In these instances there is an inexpensive and beautiful way to reduce the toxic vapors in your indoor environment - house plants!

Just as forests and jungles improve the air quality of our planet, house plants improve the air quality of your house! *How To Grow Fresh Air* lists 50 house plants that purify the air. They are rated in four categories: removal of chemical vapors, ease of growth and maintenance, resistance to insect infestation, and transpiration rate. The top ten house plants from that book (by overall rating) are: 1) Areca Palm; 2) Lady Palm; 3) Bamboo Palm; 4) Rubber Plant;
5) Dracaena "Janet Craig"; 6) English Ivy; 7) Dwarf Date Palm; 8) Ficus Alii;
9) Boston Fern; and 10) Peace Lily.

It is possible to **lower** the chemical off-gassing of new furnishings by allowing them to off-gas before bringing them indoors. You can do this by leaving them in a warm garage or on a porch for at least a few months (the longer the better) before bringing them inside. My favorite way to feel safe about furnishings (and save money too) is to obtain used furnishings!

Manufactured homes (aka mobile homes) are sold under different liability laws than site built homes. This does not mean that the chemical vapors are different. The following is a health warning that comes with manufactured homes: "Important Health Notice. Some of the building materials used in this home emit formaldehyde. Eye, nose, and throat irritation, headache, nausea, and a variety of asthma-like symptoms, including shortness of breath, have been reported as a result of formaldehyde exposure. Elderly persons and young children, as well as anyone with a history of asthma, allergies, or lung problems, may be at greater risk. Research is continuing on the possible long-term effects of exposure to formaldehyde.

Reduced ventilation resulting from energy efficiency standards may allow formaldehyde and other contaminants to accumulate in the indoor air. Additional ventilation to dilute the indoor air may be obtained from a passive or mechanical ventilation system offered by the manufacturer. Consult your dealer for information about the ventilation options offered with this home.

High indoor temperatures and humidity raise formaldehyde levels...

If you have any questions regarding the health effects of formaldehyde, consult your doctor or local health department."

There is a wonderful alternative to a conventional house and the chemical cocktail it likely contains. Recently there has been a resurgence of building homes from natural materials. Strawbale, adobe and cob are coming into vogue in many places, and if built correctly, they don't off-gas at all.

The following article entitled, *The Natural Home*, was written by Christina L. Ott (www.Barefootbuilder.com).

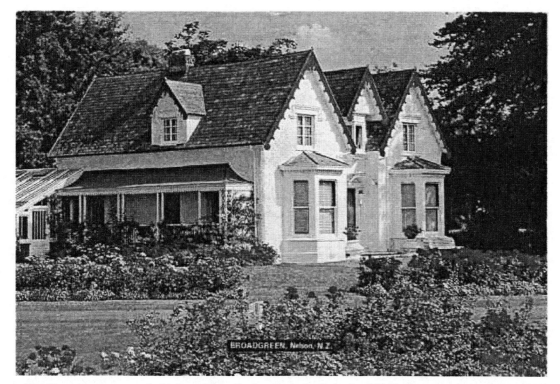

The Broadgreen estate in Nelson, New Zealand was built in the 1800's from a mixture of sand, clay, and straw known as cob. It has survived several major earthquakes that destroyed the surrounding town.

Your home is your sanctuary, the place you go to rest and recuperate, a medium for expressing who you are and perhaps the culmination of years of hard work. Buying a home is the major achievement of many people's young lives. The house is a symbol of stability, family and prosperity and is likely to be the recipient of a great deal of your time and money spent on decoration and maintenance. You will probably spend fifteen to thirty years of your life working at a job that you may love or may loathe in order to pay your mortgage. Yet this hard won sanctuary that you so treasure may also be quietly destroying your health.

The modern home is a chemical gas chamber made of thousands of toxic synthetic materials that are dangerous to builders, homeowners, and the environment. Houses are not just made of wood and brick. They are wrapped in plastic and Styrofoam painted with toxic paints, have tiles glued down with adhesives, vinyl flooring, Formica countertops, plastic carpets, formaldehyde soaked insulation, fire retardant synthetic furniture, poly-vinyl-chloride water pipes, plastic bathtubs and enameled metal ones; the list goes on and on. In fact, probably the majority of the components of a home are toxic. The chemical off-gassing from a new house (Oh, that lovely fresh smell of a new house!) can last for the entire lifetime of the building, which in the case of most homes built today is only about 50 years. At the end of that time the house becomes toxic waste, nothing more than a disposal problem for your children. Compounding the problem is the fact that well intentioned efforts at improving energy efficiency have meant that most homes now are virtually hermetically sealed. Very little fresh air comes in and few toxic chemicals can escape.

Most homes leave something to be desired in the area of human comfort as well. New homes are usually straight edged and sterile with little connection to nature. Residents often spend thousands of dollars on decorating to soften or disguise the soul impoverished linear qualities inherent to modern home design. We all come from thousands of generations of people who have lived and died surrounded by the natural environment and being surrounded in our homes by straight lines and perfectly smooth surfaces that never occur in the natural world can be subtly unsettling. Living as we do now in cities and suburbs, the closest most of us get to our ancestral environment is a chemical drenched lawn or a city park. While we may enjoy the stimulation of this lifestyle, the lack of connection with our natural environment can cause constant low level stress and ultimately damage the psyche as well as the physical body.

There is an alternative to living in a toxic synthetic environment. People built breathtakingly beautiful and comfortable homes for thousands of years before sheetrock, latex paint, fiberglass and all the rest were ever invented. Many people today are looking to these ancient traditions of architecture to provide relief from chemical induced illness and refuge from high stress environments. Houses can be built entirely from stone, wood, straw bales and earth without any synthetic materials at all. When we surround ourselves with the elements that we have evolved with throughout human history we are far less likely to be harmed by them than by chemicals that have existed only for the past two or three generations.

Earth is the oldest and most common building material on earth. About one half of the world's people live in homes built of the earth and many of us who have not grown up with these traditional buildings are beginning to see the need to revive them in the Western world. Earthen buildings in one form or another have been built for thousands of years all over the world, in Africa, Europe, Asia, and the Americas. Parts of the Great Wall of China are built from earth as well as large parts of the first great cities, Babylon and Ur. In Yemen there are cob buildings five stories high built in the middle ages and still inhabited today. In Southern England tens of thousands of cob (earthen) homes between 500 and 700 years old remain in use today as hundreds of new ones are being built with the encouragement of the Queen.

In North America there is the Taos Pueblo, the oldest constantly inhabited buildings in the U.S., built entirely from earth. Even in the northeastern US many colonial era homes are built of earth, most of the wooden ones having long ago burned or rotted away. There are at least forty adobe homes in New York over 100 years old. There are cob and adobe homes in Pennsylvania and Massachusetts. Even Paul Revere's home in Boston is built of adobe bricks.

Types of earthen building include adobe, rammed earth, wattle and daub, and cob.

Cob is a style of earthen building developed in the harsh wet environs of the British Isles. It is similar to adobe, being made of the same natural ingredients, but where adobe is formed into bricks and sun dried cob is applied directly to the foundation by the handful or by the shovelful to create hand sculpted free flowing walls. Building with cob is a creative experience similar to sculpting with clay. Cob is stronger than adobe and more resistant to wet weather because it has a higher straw content and because it is monolithic. In other words, cob is not made into individual bricks, but rather the whole building is one single brick. There are no seams for the walls to crack along.

Cob homes can be built entirely from natural materials from the foundations to the paints. These houses are cool in summer and warm in winter because of their thick walls and thoughtful designs, so they may never need to be heated or air-conditioned except in the most extreme climates. I spoke recently with a woman who grew up in a stately old adobe house in Central America. She recalled afternoon naps as a child, taken to escape murderously hot afternoons, in the pleasantly cool bedroom of her parents' thick walled earthen home.

One of the greatest benefits of a cob home is that not only will it not be poisoning you, but it can also be very inexpensive. Thus you can spend less time in a stressful work environment and more time participating in the life of your family and community which will certainly also keep you healthier and happier.

To learn more about cob homes visit www.BareFootBuilder.com, www.NaturalBuildingNetwork.org, www.CobCottage.com, www.CobWorks.com, www.DirtCheapBuilder.com.

In 1872, J. R. Black M.D. authored, *The Ten Laws of Health*. The first law in that book he called, '*Breathing a Pure Air, its Violation, and Results*'. He recommends that we keep our windows open for ventilation no matter how hot or cold the weather. The following quotes come from that book. "The foolish fear of gentle currents, even when the body is well protected, is very fruitful in mischief. It induces men and women to sit and sleep in closed, almost air tight, apartments, enveloped by an atmosphere deficient in oxygen, every inch of it abounding with the foul and deleterious exhalations from the body...The true rule, and one that deserves to be universally adopted for the preservation of health during the winter season, is to *warm dwellings less and clothe the body more*. Compare the warmly-clad, healthy pioneers, with their open, barnlike houses, and the daintily-clad, pale, shivering, sickly beings who live in airtight, oven-like rooms, and the former will be found to be very rarely victims to colds, not a few of them during a long lifetime never needing the services of a physician, while the latter nearly always feel the need of medical aid. There is nothing cheaper or more easily obtained than good, pure air; and the idea of having it foul in order to preserve its warmth, is not only sickening, but is, besides, the very worst kind of economy."

Kristine Nolfi provides modern day science to back up Dr. Black's previous quote in her book, *Raw Food Treatment of Cancer*. "Since we use five or six hundred quarts of air per hour we can soon exhaust the oxygen in a small room whose windows and doors are closed. We then inhale our own exhaled carbon dioxide and awaken to a heavy head in the morning."

The choice is yours, to ventilate or not to ventilate. But don't be fooled by air conditioning, most ac units recycle the same air. If your ac unit is equipped with an air exchanger, you should turn it on.

Mold is another hazard to indoor air quality and is one of the most insidiously dangerous indoor air pollutants. If you have mold growing indoors, I recommend that you take it very seriously. Airborne mold spores have been known to make some people so sick that they require hospitalization. Home furnishings and even walls that have mold living in them are best disposed of. Even when the visible surface mold has been cleaned off, mold can survive inside and behind sheetrock walls and in furniture, only to grow again once the chemical used to clean the surface dissipates. A dehumidifier can help by keeping the humidity level low enough to prevent mold from releasing mycotoxins and health-affecting spores. There are specially designed air purification machines that kill airborne mold spores. A company called EcoQuest manufactures these machines.

Dust mites are the most common allergen-producing organism found in our homes. They live in carpets, mattresses, upholstered furniture, and those areas that rarely get cleaned and accumulate dust. They require periods of relative humidity above 55 percent in order to thrive and breed. Keeping the humidity below 55 percent with a dehumidifier is helpful in controlling these microscopic animals.

New Car Smell

Have you ever experienced drowsiness after riding in a new car with the windows shut tight? It could be the air quality inside the passenger compartment causing your drowsiness.

New cars are a major source of volatile organic chemicals (VOCs). Most of the VOCs leach from glues, paints, plastic, and vinyl in the passenger compartment. Some people experience sore throats, nausea, headaches, and drowsiness from breathing them. Prolonged exposure can lead to much more serious heath conditions. A study done by Australia's Commonwealth Scientific and Industrial Research Organization in 2001, found that new car riders are subject to toxic emissions several times higher than the limit deemed safe for humans. Japanese car manufacturers are the first (to my knowledge) to set an industry-wide goal of reducing VOC concentrations (aka new car smell). Toyota spokesman Paul Nolasco said, "Cutting down on the things that lead to these smells is only something that can be better for you." In 2005, Toyota agreed to cut passenger compartment levels of 13 chemicals, including formaldehyde and styrene, by the year 2007. They will attempt to match Japanese Health Ministry guidelines for air quality in homes. Some of Japan's top five car manufacturers Toyota, Honda, Nissan, Mazda and Mitsubishi are already producing cars with lower VOC levels in Japan. However, in March of 2008 I contacted Toyota and Honda dealers in the USA and was told that a low VOC car was not available.

Unfortunately, the Alliance of Automobile Manufacturers, which represents nine carmakers including General Motors, Chrysler, and Ford, said in 2005, it does not follow the issue of volatile organic compounds.

If you are forced to ride in a new car and breathe the chemical cocktail, I suggest the following. Set the ventilation control to bring outside air into the car and leave the windows partially or fully open. The best solution is to drive an older car that has already off-gassed most of its chemicals.

Sunlight: The Great Healer

The USA's Environmental Protection Agency's (EPA) advice to avoid sunlight is believed by many to be based on junk science. *The Townsend Letter* (the examiner of medical alternatives), January 2004, explains why in an article entitled, *The Healing Power of Full Spectrum Lighting.*

"The phobia arose after investigators anaesthetized animals, propped their eyes open and shined intense UV light into them; this damaged their retinas. Excessive exposure to one kind of ultraviolet (short wave, germicidal UVC) can damage tissue. But the EPA makes the ridiculous leap from that truth to the conclusion that we should avoid all UV. UVC is not present increasingly in sunlight...In fact, trace amounts of UV radiation in natural daylight are required for physical and mental health, civilized behavior, muscle strength, energy, and learning.

Sunlight in moderation improves immunity and stimulates our metabolism while decreasing food craving and increasing our intelligence. Those words were taken from the book *Sunlight* by Zane R. Kime, M.D., M.S., where he backs this statement up with scientific research.

Brian Clement, Director of the Hippocrates Institute, says that sunlight is the most powerful booster of the immune system that he is aware of.

In his book, *Sunlight,* Dr. Kime explains the link between nutrition and sunburn. "Unless one has proper diet, sunlight has ill effects on the skin. This must be emphasized: sunbathing is dangerous for those who are on the standard high-fat American diet or do not get an abundance of vegetables, whole grains, and fresh fruits. Those on the standard high-fat diet should stay out of the sun and protect themselves from it; but at the same time they will suffer the consequences of both the high-fat diet and the deficiency of sunlight." Dr. Kime also summarizes several excellent studies which conclude that sunlight is a much better source of vitamin D (which more closely resembles a hormone) than the kind added to enriched foods, especially cow's milk.

My personal experience supports Dr. Kime's thesis. Before I changed my eating habits from the Standard American Diet (SAD) to the health- promoting lifestyle that I practice today, I could not spend much time in the sun without sunscreen or I would become sunburned. Ever since my positive lifestyle change, I have been able to spend as much time as I wish in full sun, without sunscreen, and never burn! After researching the matter, I found that an increased dietary intake of vitamins and other nutrients, and an avoidance of free-radical forming foods, has been scientifically shown to have that effect on humans.

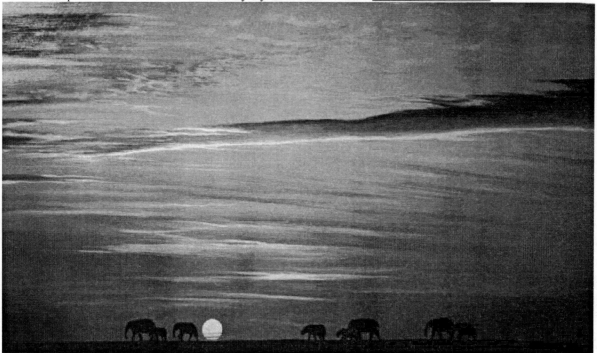

Chew, Chew, Chew!

The importance of thoroughly chewing your food cannot be overemphasized! Digestion starts in the mouth. The mouth is the first part of our digestive tract. If you do not chew your food completely, the nutrients in your food might exit the other end of your body without being absorbed. Most people say "You are what you eat" but nutritionists usually say, "You are what you absorb."

One of my favorite quotes on this topic is "Chew your liquids and drink your solids." In other words, mix your liquids with your saliva by chewing them and chew your solid food until it turns into liquid.

If you are prone to gobbling your food, try putting down the fork or spoon between each bite and not picking it up again until the mouth is empty. It is difficult to fully enjoy your food unless you eat it slowly. Appreciate the fragrance and colors of each piece of food before you put it into your mouth. Enjoy the subtle flavors and texture of the food before you swallow it. The benefits of this style of eating can have a profoundly positive effect on your digestion and ultimately your health!

Proper Rest

I suggest that we always go to sleep on an empty stomach. The body uses the time that we sleep to perform routine maintenance. Our liver must process countless amounts of dead cells and hormones that are constantly being replaced. (The liver must also deal with all the chemicals that we breath in, absorb through our skin, and consume daily.) If we eat before bed, the liver must process the food that we have just eaten and maintenance functions must wait. This may mean longer sleep time is required to feel well rested.

If you feel hungry before bed, try drinking a tall glass of water. The body will sometimes send hunger pangs when dehydrated, and a glass of water may be the fix.

Going to sleep on an empty stomach can go a long way toward waking up feeling refreshed in the morning.

Deep Relaxation

Research has led me to believe that the most beneficial position for deep relaxation is lying on your back with your arms by your sides, palms facing up, legs straight out, and toes pointing to the sides. Your breathing is deep but relaxed and the **mind is relaxed** as well as the physical body.

Studies have shown that for most people, only three months of 20 minutes per day spent in deep relaxation causes blood pressure to normalize, overall energy to increase, moods to improve, sleep to improve and both hands and feet to become warmer. This result suggests that relaxation improves circulation.

Deep relaxation can be done in bed for ten minutes upon waking in the morning and for ten minutes before going to sleep. If something happens to stress you out at any time during the day, relaxing deeply can truly help.

Weight Normalization

If you found an age-old and scientifically based method of eating that would almost effortlessly allow your weight to normalize, and if the side effects were that it would slow down your aging process, your blood pressure would normalize, your arteries would open up, your arthritis would go away, your chronic migraines would cease, your diabetes would vanish, your depression would lift and your self-esteem and energy levels would soar, would you do it? I have witnessed all of these things happening to people when they shift to a raw and living foods diet.

It is said that there are two general categories of people: those who pass all the artificial chemicals that have been consumed out the opposite end from where they came in (the skinny ones), and those who hold on to all the chemicals consumed (people who suffer from overweight). The body surrounds these chemicals with fat to protect our tissues from them. What kind of chemicals are we talking about? They are: food additives such as artificial colors, preservatives, flavor enhancers, pesticides, toxins such as acrylamide and others created from cooking, artificial sweeteners, antibiotics, growth hormones and other chemicals in animal products– literally thousands of compounds. Over the years artificial chemicals can build up in the fatty tissue and contribute to weight gain and obesity. A friend of mine once said, "If you consume bizarre laboratory-concocted nonsense, you will become bizarre laboratory-concocted nonsense." My advice is to avoid these chemicals as you would avoid a plague!

Low oxygen levels can also lead to an overweight condition. In order for the cells in our bodies to burn all the fuel that we absorb from our food, enough oxygen must be present. If sufficient oxygen is not present, unburned fuel may be stored as fat. Thus, people who take short, shallow breaths rather than long, deep ones are not using the full capacity of their lungs and may become deficient in oxygen. The lack of a sufficient amount of oxygen may be causing a buildup of unburned food to be stored as fat. See the sections entitled "Oxygen/Deep Breathing," "Deep Relaxation," and "Circulation" earlier in this chapter for more details on this subject.

Dairy products are another culprit that can contribute to an overweight condition. Cow's milk is loaded with naturally occurring growth hormones designed to turn a calf into a cow very quickly. Even organic milk contains growth hormones that can cause humans to gain weight, and non-organic dairy products have added synthetic growth hormones as well, which make them even worse. No animal consumes the milk of another species in nature, nor does any animal drink the milk of its own species as an adult. Our society has been sold on the completely false idea that cow's milk is an essential part of a healthy diet by a **paid advertising agency** called the American Dairy Council. The facts are that cow's milk causes weight gain in humans as well as in baby cows, that it is unnecessary for human health, and in large amounts is detrimental to the health of humans.

Eating living foods, provided that you keep the sweet fruits to a minimum, keeps blood sugar levels normal. When blood sugar is elevated, the pancreas floods the bloodstream with insulin, which then turns the sugars into fat. When insulin spikes, signals are sent to stop the conversion of fat to be burned for fuel. Insulin also suppresses the thyroid, which in turn slows the metabolic rate. It is well known that blood sugar elevates when we eat sugary desserts, but some people are unaware that when we eat bread and pasta, rice, potatoes and many other starchy cooked foods, and almost all processed foods, these foods also turn into simple sugars. Even products labeled as whole wheat raise insulin levels and are turned into fat.

When eating living foods, one can usually eat as much as one desires, and if overweight, one will still lose weight! It will not happen as fast as if your body went into ketosis (the biological condition induced by high-protein diets), but ketosis can be dangerous. Many people who come to see me who have been on ketosis-inducing diets start to experience panic attacks, smell like rotting flesh, and have a complexion akin to a corpse. These diets do cause you to lose weight, but eventually you gain it back, plus a few or more, pounds, and it becomes harder and harder to keep the weight off in the long run.

Dr. Robert O. Young has been helping people to normalize their weight through balancing the over-acid conditions that exist in many of his clients' bodies. He says that a fat problem can actually be an acid problem. The body maintains fat to neutralize the acid, so as you start alkalizing the tissues, the fat comes off. (See "Acid-Alkaline Balancing" in the beginning of this chapter.)

Another thing that you want to do in order to lose weight is to speed up your metabolism. The only safe way to achieve this is to eat often. Metabolism becomes slow if you skip meals like many people do when they try to lose weight. The slowing of the metabolic rate is an important evolutionary adaptation that animals, including humans have developed as a basic survival strategy. If food is scarce, the body perceives starvation, sensing that little food is coming in, or that a long time elapses between meals. To make sure there is enough fuel to keep you alive, your body stores as much of the food as it can as fat, and slows the rate at which it burns calories. Once metabolism slows down, it is extremely difficult to lose weight. The key is to eat often; but remember, it must be nutrient-dense foods. Your body will have no choice but to eventually turn up the metabolic rate and the pounds will come off! Try to eat only living foods unless you experience a healing crisis at an inappropriate time. (Be sure to read "Cleansing Reactions/The Healing Process" earlier in this chapter.) Even small amounts of processed or cooked food can slow down the weight-loss process.

To increrase the metabolic rate, I recommend five medium-sized meals a day, but don't eat before retiring for the night. Nighttime is the period when your body renews itself; the digestive organs need a 'time-out." If your body spends the first part of the night digesting food, it might not have enough time to perform the routine but essential maintenance functions.

Identical twins with different diets pictured below.

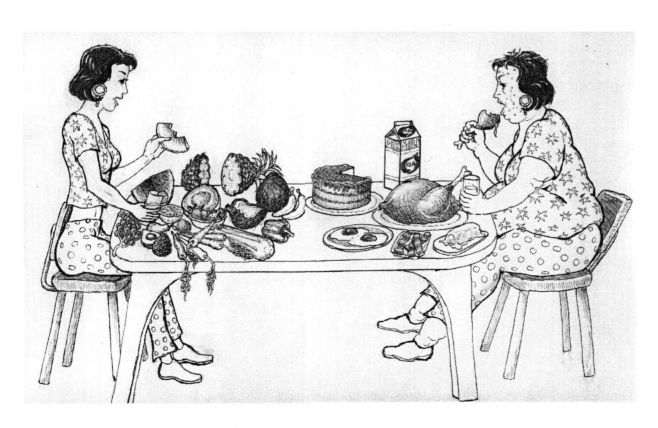

If you were considering a high protein diet, I suggest you do more research before rushing into such a dangerous diet. In an article that appeared in the August 2004 issue of *National Geographic* entitled "Why Are We So Fat?," one nutrition expert hissed, "I want to know why Atkins didn't have himself autopsied so we could see for ourselves what his coronary arteries looked like." The article goes on to say, "Atkins gets into trouble when he says to eat bacon and go into ketosis. It's a toxic state...You can lose weight in ways that aren't good for you. Smoking causes you to lose weight, as does amphetamines. But it's not just about losing weight, it's losing weight in a way that is helpful. There are no long term studies to support this diet."

When a pregnant woman craves a certain food, it is usually because she is craving a nutrient that she is lacking. Have you ever noticed that sometimes after consuming a large amount of cooked food, your stomach feels full or distended, but you are still hungry? Well what has most likely happened is that your body is craving a certain nutrient (or several) just like the pregnant woman, and is telling your brain to eat more hoping to obtain that nutrient. In Chapter One I have listed facts from the medical dictionary on vitamin loss and also information on mineral and protein loss from cooking. Next time try an organically grown raw meal and see if you are still hungry after eating it. You might also find that snacking on cut vegetables, such as celery and carrots, or fruit, such as apples and oranges, will satisfy your urges for nibbling, especially if they are fresh and organically grown, which usually have a much higher nutrient density and can be very filling.

If you stick to a healthy, mostly raw food diet, before you know it, your taste buds will change and the unhealthy foods that once tasted good to you will become unpalatable. You will be able to taste the rancidity of fried foods and wonder how you ever could have enjoyed them. You will notice how a large meal of cooked food robs your energy while raw meals leave you feeling energetic and light. The healthy foods that you once shunned will become delicious! You will even crave foods such as fresh fruits and berries, uncooked vegetables, raw nuts and seeds, sprouts and sprouted grains!

Are you aware that sometimes the body will tell you to feed it when actually it is dehydrated? If you experience hunger pangs at times when you have not had any water in a half hour or more, try drinking a cup of pure water. You might be surprised by how effective this method can be at putting a halt to unwanted nibbling.

Did you know that it can take up to 15 minutes after the stomach is full for your brain to send signals to the conscious mind informing you of its fullness? That is one of the many reasons why you should chew each bite of food very well (see the chapter entitled, "Chew, Chew, Chew"). Put down the eating utensil or piece of food between each bite and don't pick it up again until the mouth is empty. The more rapidly you eat, the more food you may ingest without realizing that you are full, only to feel bloated a few minutes later.

A high-fiber diet is very helpful in weight loss. A high-fiber meal creates a feeling of fullness and a sense of satisfaction after a meal (refer to "Fiber" in chapter one), thus helping to ward off the urge to eat again soon after a meal.

Remember that all unprocessed plant foods are high in fiber and that no animal foods contain fiber.

I would like to leave you with this thought to ponder: Have you ever seen animals in the wild on their natural living foods diet that are overweight? It just doesn't happen. The only animals that become overweight are the ones fed devitalized, processed, chemical-laden, acid-forming foods by humans. Remember, being in control of your diet means that you must consciously break old harmful habits and form new healthy ones. An 'old dog' can learn new tricks!

Use It or Lose It

In this section we will be speaking about two things: your mind and your body. By keeping them active, one will keep them functioning properly. But if we don't use our mind or our body regularly, such as in *couch potato syndrome-*where one sits in front of a television for hours on end and does not exercise the body or mind, we can lose function gradually over time. This results in a stiff and unhealthy body and a weak mind.

First let us talk about the mind. Before the year 2000 science told us that we are born with a full set of neurons (brain cells) and that we do not produce any new ones during our lifetime. Fred Gage from the Salk Institute in La Jolla, California proved that **adult humans can grow new brain cells**. He also found that physical exercise is one of the best ways to achieve this. Neurogenesis (the birth of new brain cells) is still a controversial topic in some circles, but Fred Gage's work proves that neurogenesis is a lifelong process. The controversy shall soon pass in the same way that the belief that the earth was flat was proved false just a few hundred years ago.

Research has also shown that the connections between neurons form throughout life. Neurons release chemicals called neuro-transmitters into the connections between brain cells (called synapses) to communicate with each other and the rest of our body. If we don't us these pathways often, they can become impassable. Visualize a path through a jungle. If that path is not maintained, it will become impassable. But if we frequent the path, we keep that pathway open.

The key to keeping and/or strengthening our cognitive functions (mind) is to perform mental workouts regularly. The main areas that we should work on are memory, concentration, and communication at the very least. When we learn new things, whether it is physical coordination or purely mental, our brains can add more neurons to store the new information. We can improve our cognitive functions in a more stimulating and enjoyable way when we are faced with challenging events and new ideas, such as how to improve our diet and lifestyle. The challenges that life brings us can be seen as opportunities to for self improvement.

As most people know, it is also important to continue stretching and exercising our bodies as we age. When we are children our bodies are very flexible, but as we age and stop being as active, we lose the flexibility that was once ours. Over time stiffening becomes worse and worse. By middle age, I notice that some people walk more like penguins than people. The good news is that you need not go this route! If you are still flexible, all it takes is a minimum of 20 minutes per day of carefully designed stretching. I am not speaking about putting your foot behind your head or forcing your body in any way. What I am talking about is gently stretching every part of your body: your fingers, toes, arms, legs, neck, and especially your torso. I have heard it said that **you're only as old as your spine is flexible,** and I believe that there is some truth to this statement. Keeping your spine and your entire body flexible, can and will improve the quality of your life dramatically.

After years of studying and practicing almost every modern form of 'yoga type' exercise routine, and taking two teacher trainings, one in Hatha yoga and one in Kundalini yoga, I have designed a stretching routine called *Essene Yoga*. There are no standing postures in *Essene Yoga* and it can be practiced by people of all levels of fitness, the very 'fit' person as well as the elderly. *Essene Yoga* was designed to stretch every part of the body and leave you feeling energized and not tired, as many modern types of yoga/exercise sometimes do. There are two different sets on the DVD, one that is 20 minutes long and one that is one hour long.

For those who cannot spare 20 minutes a day, I have also designed an excellent exercise DVD called *Chair Yoga for Busy People*. This DVD was designed for my 80+ year old parents. All of the exercises on the *Chair Yoga* DVD are done while sitting in a chair! There are 3 sets to choose from, including one as short as 3 minutes.

Consider this, if you do some type of stretching exercise for at least a few minutes every day, chances are that a year from now you will be more flexible and less prone to injury. But if you don't do any type of stretching exercise, chances are that a year from now you will be a bit stiffer and more prone to injury. The way that I suggest insuring that you do some type of exercise every day is to do it as soon as you get up in the morning. I know that if I put my exercise routine off until later in the day, chances are that I'll never end up doing it that day. The choice is yours. You may visit www.rawfoodsbible.com to order the exercise DVD of your choice or find a routine that works for you.

By adding some type of gentle stretching to your daily routine, and simple mind exercises, such as adding the prices of the groceries up in your head as you shop or engaging in stimulating conversation, you can keep both your mind and body fit. These healthy habits can improve the quality of your life significantly.

The Mind-Body Connection

Emotions have been scientifically proven to have a powerful effect on the immune system. Researchers in medical schools in the United States and other countries have discovered that immune cells such as T-cells, B-cells and macrophages, known as the white blood cells, have receptors for neuropeptides. Neuropeptides are created in our body every time we have a thought, and our immune cells listen for and react to the emotional dialog. Positive thoughts such as love, joy, happiness, forgiveness, and so forth, create health-promoting neuropeptides that boost the immune system, while negative thoughts such as fear, hate, jealousy, possessiveness, and so forth, create neuropeptides that can depress the immune system and lead to disease.

Negative emotions have also been shown to cause acidity in the tissues while positive emotions create alkalinity in them.

Tony Buzan explains in his cassette program, *Brain Power*, "There are thousands of documented studies of people who have recovered from illness simply through the power of the mind." He goes on to say, "Children can make themselves ill, and give themselves nose bleeds merely at the thought of an upcoming test" and, "Many people give themselves rashes in stressful situations."

Dr. Richard Anderson, N.D., N.M.D., states in book one of *Cleanse & Purify Thyself:* "Another factor in the ability to adapt a raw-food diet is emotions. Remember, thoughts and feelings are the primal directive forces that control our bodies; this includes appetites and desires. Some people will never be raw-fooders until they have transmuted certain emotions."

Stress has been scientifically proven to cause many health problems due to its effects on the nervous system. A few of these problems include insomnia, poor digestion, a weakened immune system and cellular repair system. Stress dulls the sense of touch, lowers IQ, can be a factor in cancer and heart attacks, and makes people generally meaner.

If you could only remember one thing from this book, I suggest you remember this: If there is someone in your life towards whom you feel animosity and refuse to forgive, you are not hurting them, you are hurting yourself. Forgive them and your health will benefit. I once heard someone say that holding a grudge against someone is like drinking poison and expecting the other person to die.

Many researchers are now convinced that our emotional state is just as important as our nutritional state in the quest for optimum health.

My Typical Menu

People often ask me what I eat in a typical day, so I have included this section. The first thing on my menu is not food for my body but for my spirit. Yogic type stretching in a relaxed meditative state is very healthy and should be done on an empty stomach. Even if I have to get up very early, I will get up even earlier to have time to stretch. This has been shown by researchers to lubricate joints with synovial fluid and it makes me feel great! Remember, "Use it or lose it!"

The first thing that passes my lips after water is fruit. Fruit is easy to digest compared to most other foods and it is rich in pure water and loaded with nutrients. Fruit is the original fast food and the best food to break a fast! I usually make a smoothie with a mixture of berries such as blueberries (the only food scientifically shown to reverse the aging process), raspberries, blackberries and strawberries and sometimes a banana. These berries are known to be among the richest of all foods in antioxidants. I also add barley green powder, flax seed powder, non-GMO lecithin granules, and acerola cherry powder (see Nature's Antioxidant Blast in the Recipe section).

For lunch, I usually eat vegetables with raw nuts and/or seeds. The vegetables may include carrots, celery, bok choy, tomatoes, radish, romaine lettuce, parsley, napa cabbage, broccoli, red pepper, sprouts of all kinds, arugula and zucchini. If I am on the go, I eat them whole, sometimes dipping them into raw, unsalted nut butter or guacamole. If I am in an appropriate situation, I might cut the vegetables up and toss a salad with cold-pressed, extra-virgin olive oil or an avocado whipped in the blender with water for dressing.

An afternoon snack might be sea vegetables such as dulse or bullwhip kelp, a coconut, some olives or a handful of raw pumpkin seeds or Brazil nuts.

Dinners vary and usually begin with a large salad with homemade dressing or fresh lemon juice and Essene bread with avocado or pate. Other dinners include spiralized vegetables with living marinara, curried vegetables, raw veggie-burgers, a sea vegetable dish or nori rolls (chopped vegetables on raw nori paper with avocado, or nut pate inside) and unpasteurized miso soup (served room temperature) with finely chopped vegetables in it. Recipes for all these dishes can be found in the Recipe section at the back of this book.

I occasionally take a Vitamin B12 supplement in the sublingual form (dissolving a tablet under the tongue) just to be on the safe side and I recommend this to you as well. Even people who eat foods high in B12 can become deficient in this very important vitamin due to the lack of an acid secretion in our gut called intrinsic factor. A B12 lozenge dissolved in the mouth and absorbed under the tongue into the blood steam will insure an adequate intake of B12.

Since we are all different, what works for me might not work for you. This diet works best for me. It has for many years, and I've never felt better in my life!

Summation

Cooked and processed foods are certainly able to sustain life in humans. However, unless the genetic inheritance of the person is exceptionally good, a diet high in cooked and processed foods can lead to a slow but progressive degeneration of cells and tissues which encourages early aging and the development of degenerative diseases. A living-foods diet will not make you fat and it encourages your body to reach its ideal weight.

Cooking foods can result in a 70 to 80 percent loss of vitamins, approximately a 50 percent loss of protein and a total loss of enzymes. An enzyme-deficient diet may be responsible for reduction in brain weight and size, unfavorable enlargement of the pancreas, wasting of the precursors of metabolic enzymes, and many degenerative trends.

When heated, essential fats change and can produce free radicals. Trans fats block cell respiration and are linked to cell damage and disease. New research reveals that cooked starchy foods like chips, corn products, potatoes and bread produce a highly carcinogenic chemical called acrylamide, known to cause cancer in laboratory animals. The higher the heat, the more acrylamide is formed.

It is now proven that we do not need to consume animals or their milk or eggs, and that these foods can actually cause ill heath if eaten in excess or prepared by certain methods. A diet based on a good variety of whole, uncooked, unprocessed plant foods will supply all the nutrition we need. Eating living, chemical-free plant foods encourages optimal health because of the increased antioxidant, vitamin and nutrient profile which helps to eliminate free radicals and the damage that they cause. A living foods diet also decreases the burden of dealing with toxic chemicals that cause free radical damage.

Proper nutrition is not the only health inducing factor; lifestyle, environment, and thought processes all play major rolls in the quest for optimum health.

Woman Meditating by Hector Jara

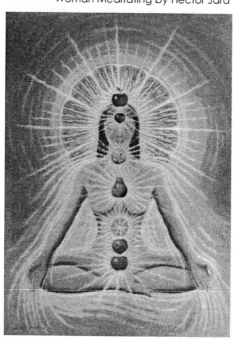

Chapter 8: Recipes

Preface to Recipes

Have you noticed the difference in taste between an organically grown, vine-ripened tomato and a genetically modified tomato? One is grown for flavor and the other is grown for shelf-life. Or the difference in taste between an extra fatty organic Hass avocado at its peak of ripeness compared to a low fat avocado? Carrots can vary in flavor from sweet to bitter, and can make a huge difference in a dish.

If you prepare a recipe with cheap ingredients, you will usually get an inferior-tasting dish. However when high quality organic ingredients are used a superior-tasting final product will be the result. I recommend tasting the ingredients before adding them into the mix.

A number of factors can cause a good recipe to come out tasting bad. Cayenne powder is available in different heat units. In one store I found two types of cayenne side by side, one contained 20,000 heat units and the other 180,000 heat units. The chefs in this book did not specify the heat units for the cayenne in their recipes. So, adding a small amount at a time and tasting the mix may be a better procedure than adding the suggested amount, and risking making the dish too hot to eat.

Stevia extract comes in different strengths, and using too much can make a recipe taste awful. Stevia that contains 90% glucosylsteviosides is much stronger than an extract of 80%. Similarly, raw honey can range in sweetness from very to mildly sweet.

Raw nuts can go rancid and should be stored in a cool place or be refrigerated. I often come across rancid macadamia and Brazil nuts in bulk bins. Although most nuts can tolerate being stored at room temperature, especially the ones with brown skins like almonds and hazelnuts, I recommend tasting all raw nuts for freshness before leaving the store.

If using unprocessed sea salt when a salt grinder is not available, I soak the salt crystals in a small amount of water and then add the water to the recipe once the salt has dissolved.

The dehydration temperatures and times listed for these recipes will vary according to the humidity and temperature of your house. Dehydration is not as specific as cooking, so don't worry about setting your alarm clock! The worst thing that can happen is that you get extra crispy food.

While experimenting with these recipes, I have found that they will usually come out tasting a bit different every time due to variations in the natural ingredients. If you are missing an ingredient or two, and you really want to prepare the recipe, I encourage you to improvise! Just go for it!

Matt Samuelson, an outstanding raw foods chef, contributed the following tips on raw food preparation:

"When preparing whole foods using the recipes in this book, it is important to be aware of the variations in natural ingredients. These recipes are best used as a guide rather than an exact formula. Due to many different factors, the flavors and textures of whole, raw foods will vary. For example, berries, peaches and tomatoes will often be sweeter in the peak of their season than in the beginning, therefore, it may be necessary to add more lemon juice to the recipe and less sweetener. This example is usually appropriate with both sweet and savory recipes.

When preparing a recipe for the first time it is recommended to add stronger flavors, i.e., salty, pungent, spicy, last. More can easily be added, whereas, it's not really possible to take out too much cayenne, salt or garlic.

Another worthy consideration when preparing foods is to be aware of one's mood or state of mind. Though there is really no scientific proof, I have experienced 'the flavor' of the chef's mood. Being relaxed, present and in appreciation is much more conducive to preparing delicious foods than being frustrated, distracted, upset or anxious.

We invite you to entertain these ideas while 'playing' in the kitchen. And remember, good food transcends all boundaries."

Measurement Equivalent Chart

A pinch	1/8 tsp or less
3 teaspoons (tsp)	1 Tbsp
2 tablespoons (Tbsp)	1/8 cup (c)
4 Tbsp	1/4 cup
16 Tbsp	1 cup
5 Tbsp + 1 tsp	1/3 cup
1 ounce (oz)	2 Tbsp liquid
4 ounce	1/2 cup
8 ounce	1 cup
16 ounce	1 pound (lb)
1 cup liquid	1/2 pint
2 cups	1 pint
2 pints (pt)	1 quart (qt)
4 cups liquid	1 quart
4 quarts	1 gallon
8 quarts	1 peck (peppers, apples, etc.)
1 jigger	1½ fluid ounces (fl oz)
1 jigger	3 Tbsp

Desserts

Cakes, Cookies, Pies, Vegan Ice Cream and more!

Raw Carob Cheesecake
Makes one 8-inch diameter cheesecake, 8-16 pieces

Ingredients for crust:
2 cups pecans, soaked for 4-6 hrs. and dehydrated until dry
1/4 cup seedless raisins
1 tsp cinnamon
1/4 cup pitted dates (medjool or sticky)
1 Tbsp raw agave or raw honey or 1 packet stevia powder (do not add more stevia or a bitter taste will occur)

Ingredients for filling:
2/3 cup unrefined coconut oil (not coconut cream or coconut milk), liquefied (to liquefy, place oil jar in a pan of hot water)
1¼ cup pitted dates
1 quart raw cashews soaked at least 3 hrs. and then rinsed
1 cup raw carob powder
1 Tbsp vanilla extract
1/2 tsp cinnamon
1 Tbsp raw agave or raw honey or 1 packet stevia powder (do not add more stevia or it will cause a bitter taste)

To make the crust:
Place the pecans, raisins, dates, honey and cinnamon in a food processor and process until ingredients begin to stick together. Press crust mixture evenly into the bottom of an 8-inch spring form pan and set aside.

To make the filling:
Place the soaked and drained cashews and liquefied coconut oil in a food processor and process until semi-smooth. Add remaining ingredients and process until creamy.
Place the filling in the crust and spread evenly. Refrigerate for at least 2-3 hrs. before serving.
Lasts for 2 weeks if stored in sealed container in the refrigerator or for 2 months in the freezer.

Recipe by Cheri Soria, www.rawfoodchef.com and modified by Craig Sommers

Meyer Lemon-Lavender Cheesecake with Wild Blackberry Coulis
Serves 8

Ingredients for crust:

1 cup pecans (soak for at least 3 hours)

1 cup shredded coconut

3/8 cup pitted dates

1 Tbsp maple sugar (optional, not a raw product)

1/4 tsp Celtic sea salt

Ingredients for lemon cream:

1 2/3 cup raw cashews

1¼ cup young coconut meat (2 – 3 Thai coconuts)

2/3 cup Meyer lemon juice

6 Tbsp lavender or blackberry honey

6 Tbsp unrefined coconut oil

2½ Tbsp chopped ginger

1/2 Tbsp vanilla extract

2/3 tsp dried lavender flowers

2 Tbsp lemon zest (5 – 6 lemons if making it yourself)

Ingredients for blackberry coulis:

10 oz blackberries, fresh or frozen

3 Tbsp raw agave nectar

Ingredients for garnish:

8 – 12 shaved pecans

8 mint sprigs

Wild berries

To make crust: Place pecans, shredded coconut, dates, maple sugar and sea salt into a food processor and blend with the S blade into a fine consistency. Press pecan mixture into a 9-inch spring form pan.

To make lemon cream: In a higher speed blender, place coconut meat, lemon juice, honey, coconut oil, ginger and vanilla and blend until smooth. Add cashews and lavender and again, blend until smooth. Add lemon zest and blend on low speed. Using a spatula, remove mixture from the blender and place into the spring form pan. Place cake into the freezer for 2 hours. Thaw for approximately 10 minutes before serving.

To make blackberry coulis: Place blackberries and agave nectar into a high speed blender and blend until smooth. Strain coulis through a fine sieve or nut milk bag. Pour into a squeeze bottle.

To assemble: Using a zester, shave pecans onto cheesecake. Squeeze blackberry coulis in an artistic pattern on the plate. Place one slice of cheesecake in the center of the plate. Garnish with wild berries and a mint sprig.

Recipe by Joshua McHugh, www.livingintentions.com

Ducky Cakes
Yields approx. 15 ducks (4 oz. each)

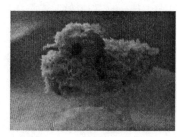

Ingredients fruit:
1 cup dried apricots
1 cup dried figs
1 cup dried apples
1 cup dried currants
1 cup dried mangos (soaked 1 hour)
1 cup pitted dates (soaked 5 hours--keep 1 cup soak water)

Ingredients nuts:
1 cup walnuts chopped (soaked 4-8 hours and rinsed)
½ cup almonds (soaked 8 hours and rinsed), peeling optional

Ingredients spices:
1 Tbsp lemon peel
1 Tbsp ginger
1 Tbsp cinnamon

Ingredients icing:
1 cup pine nuts
¼ cup freshly-squeezed lemon juice
Date water as needed for smooth consistency
2 Tbsp raw agave nectar

Ingredients other:
Coconut shavings (for duck coat)

To make icing:
Blend all icing ingredients well and chill.

To make:
Set aside one dried mango and cut into small trapezoids for duck bills.
Set aside a handful of currants for eyes.
Cut up all fruit into bite-sized pieces (except currants).
Mix all fruit with walnuts in large bowl (except mangos and dates).
Grind mangos and dates with almonds in a food processor.
Add to bowl of fruit & nuts.
Add spices and knead thoroughly.
On a large board, begin shaping 4oz. balls into duck shapes.

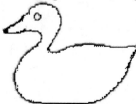

Frost with icing.
Garnish with duck bill and eyes. Add coconut shavings, covering the ducks.
Chill for a few hours. Voila! Bon Appetite!
You can adapt the recipe to make other shapes.
Recipe by Dana Pettaway, www.theraway.com

Strawberry Minicake
Yields a 6-inch minicake

Ingredients cake:
10-12 strawberries
5 or 6 pitted dates
1 tsp freshly squeezed lemon juice
½ tsp virgin coconut oil
½ cup walnuts (soaked 4-8 hours and rinsed)
½ cup raw almonds (soaked 8 hours and rinsed)
¼ cup raw agave syrup

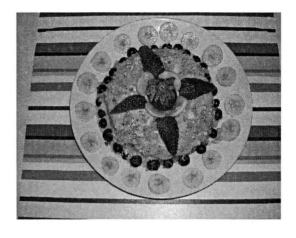

Ingredients icing:
½ cup pine nuts
¼ cup freshly squeezed lemon juice
¼ cup raw agave syrup
½ tsp vanilla extract
¼ cup raw macadamia nuts

Ingredients topping:
1 handful blueberries (frozen are ok)

Ingredients garnish:
1 banana

To make cake:
Process the nuts in a food processor and set aside. Blend dates and lemon to achieve a paste and add to processed nuts.
Set aside one strawberry and cut up the remaining strawberries. Then add the cut strawberries to the mix. Mix the contents of the bowl with your hands and form into a cake on a plate.

To make icing:
Blend all icing ingredients in a food processor except the macadamia nuts. Pour the icing over the cake and spread evenly. Process the macadamias in a food processor and sprinkle over the cake. Decorate with the blueberries and the remaining strawberry cut in 4 sections. Cut the banana into slices and garnish the plate to look like the picture. The banana slices may be dipped in lemon juice to prevent them from turning brown.

Recipe by Dana Pettaway, www.theraway.com

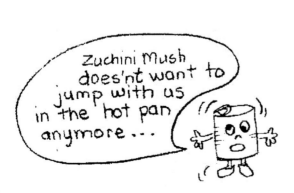

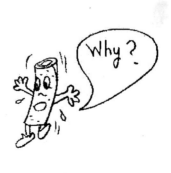

Amazing Oatmeal Carob Cookies
Makes 40 medium cookies

Ingredients:

3½ cups oat groats soaked overnight or sprouted

1 cup walnuts soaked overnight and rinsed well, then chopped

1 cup sun-dried raisins

½ cup raw carob powder

3 Tbsp raw agave, or raw honey or 2 packets stevia powder (do not add more stevia or it will cause a bitter taste)

8 oz fresh-squeezed carrot juice

2-inch piece of ginger

6 medjool dates or any sticky dates (pitted)

1 tsp unprocessed sea salt

1 tsp cinnamon powder

5 tsp unprocessed coconut oil (to liquefy, place bottle in hot water)

To make:

Juice the carrots and ginger. Process the soaked oat groats in a food processor until chopped well. Add **liquefied** coconut oil, dates, carrot-ginger juice, honey, carob powder, sea salt and cinnamon and process until all ingredients are mixed thoroughly (it might be necessary to process in small batches).

In a mixing bowl, mix contents of food processor with the raisins and chopped walnuts.

Spoon out cookie-sized amounts onto dehydrator shelves covered with nonbleached parchment paper. (Fills about 3 shelves)

Dehydrate at 100 degrees for 26 to 30 hours (less if in a dry climate) or until firm.

Refrigerate in airtight container. Yummy!

Recipe by Craig Sommers www.rawfoodsbible.com

Chokecherry Macaroons
Yields approximately 150 coin-sized cookies

Ingredients:

2 cups chokecherries or other pitted cherries, fresh or frozen

2 cups pitted dates

2 cups shredded coconut (unsweetened)

12 medium-sized apples, cored

2 cups pure water

To make:

Blend water and chokecherries in a blender. Strain out the pits if using chokecherries.

Place the cherry syrup and the cored apples in a food processor and blend using the S blade.

Mix the dates and coconut together in a food processor and combine with the apple/cherry mix.

Place Tbsp sized dollops on dehydrator sheets and dry overnight at 110 degrees.

Recipe by Katrina Blair, www.turtlerefuge.org

Apple-Oat-Nut Cookies

Ingredients:

2 cups walnuts, soaked for 2 hours
2 cups rolled oats, soaked 1 hour (old-fashioned, not instant)
2 large or 3 small Gala apples
1 large ripe banana
1 cup flame raisins
¼ tsp ground nutmeg
1 tsp vanilla extract
1 sweet tangerine, juice of

To make:

Wash and core the apples, then chop them in a food processor until shredded. Apply tangerine juice to the shredded apples and set aside. Drain and rinse the walnuts, then chop them in a food processor until they reach the consistency of chunky risotto. In a large bowl, mash the banana and then mix in the apple shreds. Drain the soaked oats and add only enough to the apple-banana mixture to reach a pleasing consistency. Add chopped walnuts and raisins while mixing until the mixture becomes a bit dry. Mix in nutmeg and vanilla.

Shape into patties about 1–2 inches across and ½ inch thick. Place on teflex or nonbleached parchment paper lined dehydrator sheets. Dehydrate at 110 degrees for 4 – 6 hours or until cookies hold together when handled.

Recipe by Terri Hix.

Butternut Squash Cookies
Makes 7-11

Ingredients:

4 cups peeled butternut squash, chopped
1 cup raisins
1 orange, juice of
½ tsp nutmeg
1 tsp cinnamon
3 Tbsp raw honey

To make:

Blend the chopped squash in a food processor using the S blade and transfer into a mixing bowl.

Blend the raisins and orange juice in the food processor. Add the raisin mixture to the squash and hand mix.

Add the rest of the ingredients into the bowl and mix thoroughly.

Flatten an ice-cream scoop-sized glob of the mixture onto a dehydrator tray until each cookie is about 1-inch thick. Set dehydrator at 100 degrees and leave for 12 - 15 hours.

Recipe by The Raw Family, www.rawfamily.com

Blueberry Pie
Yields a 12-inch pie

Ingredients for the crust:
2 cups almonds
½ cups dates, pitted and soaked
Ingredients for the filling:
5 cups blueberries
2 bananas
1½ Tbsp raw honey

To make the crust:
1. In a food processor, grind the almonds until fine.
2. Add the dates and blend until smooth.
3. Remove from processor and pat down into a pie plate.

To make the filling:
1. In a food processor, combine 4 cups of blueberries, 2 bananas, and 1½ Tbsp of raw honey. Blend until smooth.
2. Remove from food processor and add in remaining 1 cup of whole blueberries to the mix.
3. Pour into crust.
4. Refrigerate for at least 3 hours.

Note: This pie will solidify after a few hours in the fridge.

This pie has a jelled blueberry filling and mounds of whole blueberries just like traditional blueberry pie.

Recipe by Alissa Cohen, www.alissacohen.com

"Tapioca" Pudding

Ingredients:
1 cup chia seed soaked in 6-7 cups of pure water for 8 hours or longer.
1 cup raw, organic coconut flour (finely ground coconut) or shredded coconut
2-4 Tbsp raw agave nectar
1-2 tsp pure, organic, raw vanilla powder or vanilla extract
Pinch of unprocessed salt
1 tsp cinnamon powder (optional)

To make:
· Chia seed will have absorbed all of the water and expanded. It will be thick and gelatinous.
· Stir coconut flour into chia.
· Add vanilla powder, salt and cinnamon, if using.
· Stir in agave nectar. Taste, add more agave nectar if additional sweetness is desired.

This looks and tastes amazingly similar to the real thing, without all the sugar and milk!

Recipe by Dr. Ritamarie Loscalzo, www.drritamarie.com

Litchgate Sweet Potato Pie
Serves 8-16

Ingredients for crust:

2¼ cups pecans, soaked for 3 hours and rinsed

¼ cup pitted dates (soft ones)

¼ cup raisins (soft ones)

¼ tsp unprocessed sea salt

½ tsp apple pie spice (cinnamon, fenugreek, lemon peel, ginger, cloves, nutmeg)

1 pinch cayenne

Ingredients for filling:

3 cups peeled and cubed sweet potato or yam (about 1½ large potatoes)

¼ cup pitted dates (soft ones)

½ tsp freshly squeezed lemon juice

¼ tsp unprocessed sea salt

¼ tsp nonalcoholic vanilla extract

1 tsp unprocessed coconut oil

1¼ tsp apple pie spice

1 tsp raw agave syrup or raw honey or 1 packet stevia powder (do not add more stevia or it will cause a bitter taste)

To make the crust:

Place all the ingredients for the crust in a food processor, using the S blade, process until the contents begin to stick together when pinched. Press the mix into a pie plate coated with coconut oil.

To make the filling:

Place all the ingredients for the filling into a food processor, using the S blade process until smooth.

To assemble:

Pour the filling into the crust, spread evenly until smooth, draw a heart shape in the filling, chill for a few hours in the refrigerator and serve.

Recipe by Christina Ott and Craig Sommers www.rawfoodsbible.com

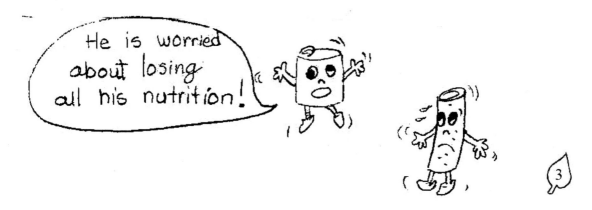

Pumpkin Pie
Serves 8–12

Ingredients for filling:

6 cups cubed (1 inch) pumpkin, no skin

1/2 cup pitted dates

2/3 cup dried apricots soaked in pure water until soft (add 1/3 cup soak water to the pie mix)

1/4 cup unprocessed coconut oil, liquefied by submerging the jar of oil in hot water

2 tsp freshly-squeezed lemon juice

1½ tsp pumpkin pie spice

1 tsp unprocessed sea salt, fine ground

1 tsp psyllium powder

Ingredients for crust:

1 cup pecans soaked overnight and rinsed

½ cup Brazil nuts, unsoaked

½ cup shredded coconut, unsweetened

½ cup pitted dates

½ tsp pumpkin pie spice

1 tiny pinch of cayenne (optional)

To make filling:

Process all the filling ingredients in a food processor using the S blade. Add one cup of pumpkin at a time and process. If they do not all fit at once, process in small batches (final mix may fit in the food processor and is suggested to insure proper mixing) Process until smooth and creamy.

To make crust:

Place all the crust ingredients in the food processor and process until the mix begins to form a ball of dough. Stop the machine if you see pieces stuck to the side and use a rubber spatula to wipe the pieces back into the mix, then process some more.

To assemble:

Press the dough into a pie pan that has been greased with coconut oil. Pour the filling in to the pie pan and refrigerate for 3 hours or more. Serve cold.

Recipe by Christina Ott and Craig Sommers, www.rawfoodsbible.com

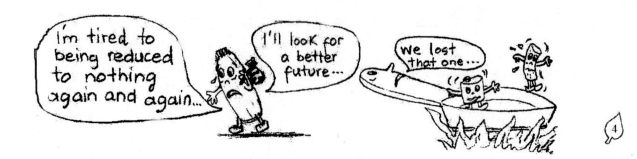

Living Banana Coconut Cream Pie
Serves 8

Ingredients for crust:

1½ cups pecans (soaked in a dark place for 8-12 hrs.)

1/2 cup pitted dates

1/2 tsp cinnamon

Ingredients for filling:

3/4 cup pitted dates

1½ cups unsweetened shredded coconut

3/4 -1 cup pure water

1/4 cup fresh-squeezed orange juice

1 Tbsp orange zest

1/8 tsp Celtic sea salt

6 medium ripe bananas

Ingredients for almond cream:

2 cups almonds (soaked 12 hours)

3/4 -1 cup water

1/4 tsp Celtic sea salt

1/3 cup pitted dates or 100% pure maple syrup (maple syrup is not raw)

1 Tbsp vanilla extract

1 Tbsp psyllium powder (optional)

To make crust:

Place all crust ingredients in a food processor and process with the S blade until the mixture sticks together when you form a ball in your hand. Press into a 9-inch glass pie plate. **Optional:** dehydrate the pecans for 12 hours after soaking or dehydrate the whole crust for 12 hours. This will give a crunchy texture to the crust.

To make filling:

With the exception of the bananas, place the rest of the ingredients for the filling in a food processor and process with the S blade until smooth.

To make almond cream:

Mix the almonds and water in a blender until creamy. Add the remaining ingredients and continue to mix until smooth (may need a food processor). For a thicker almond cream, add 1 Tbsp psyllium powder.

To assemble:

Add a thin layer of coconut filling on top of the crust. Lay 3 sliced bananas on top of that. Then add ½ the coconut filling, then ½ the almond cream. Layer 3 more bananas, the rest of the coconut filling, and the rest of the almond cream. Spread some shredded coconut on the top. Refrigerate for 2 or more hours before serving.

Recipe by Elaina Love, www.purejoylivingfoods.com

Nut-Free Banana Mango Pie
Serves 8

Ingredients for crust:

3 cups of sprouted buckwheat

1 cup shelled hempseeds (make sure they are not rancid by tasting them)

1 cup hulled sesame seeds

1 cup shredded coconut (sugar free)

2 cups pitted dates

Ingredients for filling:

2 bananas

2 very ripe mangos

½ cup unrefined coconut oil

¾ cup hempseeds

shredded coconut as needed to achieve proper density

Ingredients for topping:

Peaches

Berries (your choice)

To make crust:

Add all ingredients to a food processor and process with the S blade until the mix sticks together when pinched. Push the crust into a pie pan that has been coated with coconut oil (so that the crust doesn't stick to the pan).

To make the filling:

Add all the ingredients except the shredded coconut to a food processor and process until smooth. Start adding shredded coconut, a small amount at a time, until the mixture becomes stiff enough to spoon into the crust.

Top with berries and sliced peaches. Chill before serving.

Recipe by Tenasi Rama.

Almost Famous Apple Pie
Serves 8

Ingredients crust:

2 cups almonds (soaked 12-24 hours)

2 cups pitted dates

1 tsp orange or lemon zest

Ingredients filling:

9–12 organic apples

1 cup raisins (soaked several hours in just enough water to cover them)

2 Tbsp ground flax seeds or slippery elm powder or psyllium powder

2 tsp cinnamon powder

½ tsp allspice powder

1 pinch Garam masala

To make crust:

Place all crust ingredients in a food processor and process with the S blade until it resembles dough. Press into a pie plate.

To make filling:

Core and chop the apples into medium sized pieces. Place half the apples into a food processor along with the rest of the ingredients, including the water from the soaking raisins, and process until smooth. Set aside the mixture in a mixing bowl. Place the rest of the apples in the food processor and pulse until a chunky texture is achieved. Mix the batches together. Pour into the pie shell and enjoy! Letting the pie settle in the refrigerator for a few hours will stiffen up the filling.

Recipe by Rawsome Café / Raw for Life, www.rawforlife.com

Cranberry Apple Pie
Serves 8

Ingredients for crust:

1/2 cup dates or figs
1/2 cup raisins
1 cup Brazil nuts (soak 3 hrs and rinse)
1/2 cup shredded coconut
Dash Celtic sea salt
Dash cinnamon

Ingredients for filling:

5 Granny Smith apples
2 cups walnuts (soak for 3 hrs and rinse)
2 cups cranberries (frozen are ok)
1 tsp cinnamon
1/4 tsp nutmeg
1/3 cup golden raisins
1/3 cup raw honey
1 cup freshly-squeezed lemon juice

To make the crust:

Blend all the ingredients in a food processor until well mixed and then press it into a pie pan making an even crust.

To make the filling:

Combine the lemon juice, cinnamon, and honey. Peel and slice all the apples. Chop 4 of the apples into one-inch squares (approximately) leaving one sliced, then marinate all of them in the lemon juice mixture for 3 hours (mix well once per hour). Pulse the cranberries, walnuts and remaining honey in a food processor until a thick chunky mixture forms. Layer the apple pieces over the crust and add a layer of the cranberry-walnut mixture and half of the raisins. Continue layering until all ingredients are used. Leave the apple slices to form the very top layer (one slice per pie slice). Chill and serve!

Recipe by Shanti Devi Michal, email rawpeach25@yahoo.com

Strawberry Pie
Yields one 9-inch diameter pie

Ingredients for crust:

1 cup raisins or pitted dates
1 cup almonds, soaked overnight (dehydrate after soaking, optional)
1 cup walnuts, soaked overnight (dehydrate after soaking, optional)
1 lemon, juice of
1/3 tsp cinnamon powder
1/4 tsp clove powder
2 drops almond extract
1 tsp vanilla extract

Ingredients for filling:

1 cup raisins or pitted dates
1 banana or mango
1 pound strawberries
1 lemon, freshly-squeezed juice of
3 Tbsp psyllium husk powder

To make crust:

Place the almonds and walnuts in a food processor and mix until finely ground. While the processor is running add the dates or raisins and the remaining ingredients.

Press the pie dough into a 9 inch pie pan. Alternatively, you can roll out the crust dough with a rolling pin and use a spring form pan with the bottom removed to cut out a circle of crust that will fit inside the pan. Then place the dough on a flat plate and place the springform over it.

To make the filling:

Place the raisins or dates into a food processor and mix with lemon juice to a fine paste. Dice the strawberries and place them along with the remaining ingredients into the food processor and pulse the mix to a coarse consistency.

To assemble:

Fill the crust with the filling and refrigerate for 1 to 2 hours before serving.

Optional toppings:

Topping #1- Sweet nut sour cream topping

Ingredients for topping #1 :

1 cup raw macadamia or cashew nuts
1 lemon, freshly pressed juice of
1–2 cups pure water
3 Tbsp raw agave nectar or raw honey

To make topping #1:

Mix all ingredients in a blender until smooth. (Starting with 1 cup of water and being careful not to add too much water as to keep the topping from becoming too runny.) The pie needs 1–2 hours of chilling in a refrigerator before serving.

Topping #2- Sweet coconut cream topping

Ingredients for topping #2:

1 cup young Thai coconut meat
1 cup shredded coconut meat, sugar free
3 Tbsp raw agave nectar or raw honey

To make topping #2:
Place the shredded coconut into a blender and grind until smooth. Add the fresh coconut meat and sweetener and blend more. The pie may now be topped and then chilled before serving.

Recipe by Ursula Horaitis, www.goodmoodfood.com

Banini
Yields one blender full (smoothie)

Ingredients:
4 frozen bananas (peel before freezing)
1 fresh banana
1 tsp vanilla extract
¼ cup raw tahini
1 Tbsp maple syrup (optional)
pure water

To make:
In a blender, start with one cup pure water. Add the remaining ingredients and blend. If too thick, add more water. Suggested variations: add strawberries, carob or mint.

Recipe by Gentle World, www.gentleworld.org

Double Cacao Fudge

Ingredients:
1½ lbs dates, pitted
½ lb cacao, ground into powder with a coffee bean grinder
¼ cup coconut oil
½ teaspoon unprocessed sea salt
1 tsp raw agave

To make:
Blend all ingredients together in a food processor using the S blade.
Scoop out onto flat surface, refrigerate for a few hours until firm.
Cut into squares and serve.

Variation:
Lavender Double Cacao Fudge
Same as above - adding 1 tablespoon lavender, ground
(((Live to the point of tears)))

Recipe by Green Life Evolution Center.

Raw Medicinal Chocolate
Yields about 1½ cups

Ingredients:

1 cup ground raw cacao (powder cacao beans or nibs in a coffee bean grinder)
1/2 cup raw agave nectar
1/8 cup coconut butter, liquefied by warming (also known as coconut oil)
1/4 -1/2 cup soaked goji berries (soak for 1 hour)
1 - 2 heaping Tbsp of maca powder
1 - 2 tsp ginseng powder of choice (American or Korean)
1 pinch of Himalayan sea salt

To make:

Blend all ingredients together in a blender while calling in ancient wisdom, longevity forces and ecstatic states of bliss.

To serve:

Spread thin into dish and freeze for a fudgey experience or dip strawberries in it or drizzle onto blueberries, mango or any other fruit. Being creative with how one consumes this concoction is invited, and sharing it with loved ones is strongly encouraged.

Recipe by Heather Dunbar (aka the Chocolate Love Goddess)
www.thaistylehomestead.com

Blueberry Topping
Makes 2 cups

Ingredients:

1 pound blueberries
2 Tbsp raw honey
1-2 Tbsp ground flax seeds

To make:

Place ¾ of the blueberries in a blender with the honey and blend until smooth. Add the flax powder and blend just enough to mix well. The mixture needs time to thicken. Hand-mix the remaining whole blueberries into the mixture just prior to serving.

A coffee bean grinder works well for grinding flax seeds.

Recipe by Ananda Singh.

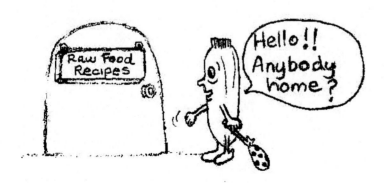

Chocolate Mousse Torte with Fresh Berries
Serves 8

Ingredients for crust:
1 cup shredded coconut
1 cup raw macadamia nuts or 1 cup soaked almonds or pecans
1/8 – 1/4 cup packed pitted dates
½ tsp Celtic sea salt
pinch of cayenne pepper
1 - 1½ tsp unprocessed coconut oil (optional for extra rich crust)

Ingredients for assembly and garnish:
Strawberries, other berries of choice, pitted cherries, and shredded coconut

Ingredients for the filling:
2 medium to large avocadoes
1 Tbsp vanilla extract
¼ tsp Celtic sea salt
3/8 – 1/2 cup raw carob powder
3/8 – 1/2 cup raw agave or raw honey

To make crust:
Place dry shredded coconut in food processor with S blade and blend into fine powder. Add nuts, salt and cayenne and blend until a texture of coarse meal is achieved. Break up dates or chop finely if very hard and distribute evenly on top of nut mixture. Homogenize until texture resembles a graham cracker crust. Mixture should be loose and crumbly and hold together when pressed lightly.

Press the crust into a 9-inch ungreased pie plate. Press firmly to get the crust to hold together. Place the crust in the freezer or refrigerator to set while making the filling.

To make filling:
Place all ingredients in food processor with S blade and homogenize until completely smooth.

To assemble:
Divide the filling into thirds. Spread a thin layer of filling in the crust. Next, place one layer of strawberries on the filling. Spread another layer of filling, then more strawberries and finish with remaining filling.

Garnish with shredded coconut, fresh berries, cherries, etc.

Refrigerate at least one hour before serving.

Recipe by Matt Samuelson, mattsamuelson@yahoo.com

Banana Ice Cream
Serves 2

Ingredients:
2 frozen ripe bananas (peel before freezing)

To make:
Process the frozen bananas with an Omega 8001, 8002 or 8003 juicer, or with a Champion juicer, using the blank plate. Serve quickly, before the bananas have time to thaw.

Recipe by Evelyn Trovinger

Pine Nut Ice Cream
Serves 2-4

Ingredients:
1 cup pine nuts
1 cup pure water
4 tsp raw agave or raw honey or maple syrup (not a raw product)
½ tsp vanilla extract
¼ tsp unprocessed sea salt

To make:
Place all ingredients in a blender and process until very smooth. Pour into a stainless steel or Pyrex bowl, seal top and freeze. Eat when frozen. Or use an old fashioned ice cream maker to freeze the mixture. Yum!

Recipe by Christina Ott, www.barefootbuilder.com

Coconut Ice Cream

Ingredients:
2 cups raw cashews soaked a minimum of 4 hours
2 cups fresh young coconut meat
1 cup coconut water
½ cup raw agave nectar
¼ cup virgin coconut oil
2 Tbsp vanilla extract
½ tsp unprocessed sea salt

To make:
Place coconut meat and water in a blender and mix until smooth. Pour mixture out of blender. Place rinsed and drained cashews in the blender and add just enough coconut mixture to cover the cashews and blend. Add the remaining ingredients to blender and process until smooth. If coconut oil is solid, liquefy by placing the jar in hot water for several minutes.

Place the mixture into a glass bowl and freeze for about 2 hours. Then add the mixture to an ice cream maker and churn.

When the ice cream is just about to the consistency desired, add chopped nuts such pecans if desired.

Enjoy!

Recipe by Shelly Nowakowski; email: shellynrawfoodie@gmail.com

Mexican "Fried" Iscream
Serves 6

Ingredients:
6 frozen bananas (before freezing, peel ripe slightly spotted bananas)
¼ tsp cinnamon (per banana)

Ingredients for Almond ice
1 cup raw almonds, soaked 12 – 24 hours, rinsed clean
2 cups of pure water
2 Tbsp of agave nectar or 3 pitted dates or 2 Tbsp of raw honey
1 tsp vanilla extract or ¼ tsp vanilla bean meat

Ingredients for caramel sauce:

1 cup pine nuts

1 cup dates, pitted

1/8 cup raw tahini (optional)

1/8 cup of unprocessed coconut oil

1/2 tsp vanilla extract or ¼ tsp of vanilla bean meat

pure water as needed to thin

dash of cinnamon to garnish each serving

To make almond ice:

Make almond milk by blending all almond ice ingredients in a blender until smooth. Strain the milk from the pulp (through a nut milk or paint strainer bag or mesh strainer), then pour the milk into the ice cube trays (2 trays each holding 12 ice cubes) and freeze.

To make Iscream:

For each serving place one frozen banana, cinnamon and 4 of the almond ice cubes in a blender (a high speed is preferable like a Vita-mix), and blend to a thick, smoothie like consistency. (Plain ice cubes can be substituted for almond ice for an Italian ice flavor instead.) You may be able to make 2–3 servings at a time, space permitting in your blender.

Set aside in the freezer until the sauce is completed.

To make caramel sauce:

Make sauce just before serving or you will need to warm the sauce in a dehydrator or in a bowl of warm water to melt to a liquid again. Blend all of the caramel sauce ingredients in the blender until smooth, adding water as needed to create a smooth sauce you can pour.

To serve:

Place one or two rounded scoops of the Iscream in each dish. Pour the caramel sauce over each scoop of Iscream and set in the freezer to harden the caramel for a few minutes. Then sprinkle the top with a dash of cinnamon, and serve.

Recipe by Kimberly Mac, www.thenakedvegan.com

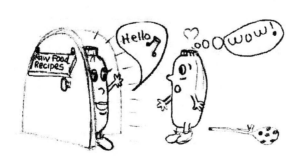

Appetizers

Pesto Stuffed Mushrooms
Yields 22 or more

Ingredients:

22 button mushrooms, washed and stemmed
1 cup walnuts, soaked several hours and rinsed
½ cup pine nuts
2 cups fresh basil
½ cup cold-pressed extra-virgin olive oil
3 cloves garlic
½ teaspoon unprocessed sea salt

To make:

1. Place mushroom caps top side down on a plate
2. Blend all stuffing ingredients (everything except the mushrooms) in a food processor until smooth.
3. Scoop a small amount of stuffing into each mushroom cap.
4. Dehydrate at 105 degrees for 5-6 hours, or until soft.

Served warm out of the dehydrator, these are heavenly! These taste like a soft, breaded, cooked, stuffed mushroom.

Recipe by Alissa Cohen, www.alissacohen.com

Durian On Fire
Serves 2-4

Ingredients:

½ medium sized durian
1 green or young Thai coconut (both water and meat)
2 ribs celery
2 ribs/leaves bok choy
1 small piece of fresh red cayenne pepper or jalapeno pepper

To make:

Cut open durian and empty half of it. Remove the pit from every piece of durian and put the yellowish meat into a blender. Remove the leaves from the celery and discard them. Chop celery and bok choy and add into blender. Add water and meat of one coconut into the blender. Add small piece of fresh red cayenne pepper or jalapeno pepper into the blender. (Note: this pepper could be very spicy so use a very small piece first. You can always add more later.) Blend everything together and serve in glasses or bowls.

Recipe by Alok, founder & director of the Alok Holistic Health center, www.alokhealth.com

Lime Pudding
Serves 2

Ingredients:
2 cups avocado
1½ cups lime, no seeds or skin
2 limes, juice of
½ cup raw agave syrup or 1 cup pitted dates (soft ones)

To make:
Process all ingredients in a food processor with the S blade.

If you love limes, this is a dream come true.

Recipe by Brigitte Mars, www.brigittemars.com

Enchanted Pistachi Vado
Serves 2

Ingredients:
1 medium-to-large sized Hass avocado
2 cups young coconut water (water will work if coconut water is not
available, but then it will not be enchanted!)
10 dates (medjool or soft)
1½ tsp vanilla extract (nonalcoholic)
2-4 Tbsp chopped pistachios (optional)

To make:
Blend everything except pistachios. Sprinkle chopped pistachios on top. For thicker pudding, add less water.

Recipe by Chad Faulk of Dazzling Earth Foods.

Shining Sushetta
Makes 1

Ingredients:
1 nori sheet
1 rib of celery
Raw nut butter of your choice
Raw honey or raw agave
Bee pollen and/or spirulina
Cucumber (optional)

To make:
Lay nori sheet flat, place celery stalk at end. Spread nut butter across stalk, drizzle honey over nut butter. Sprinkle spirulina on top, dice cucumber chunks and place on top. Wrap it up with the nori sheet and eat!

Recipe by Chad Faulk of Dazzling Earth Foods.

Live Holiday Nuts

Ingredients:
1 cup raw almonds
1 cup pecan halves
1 cup hazelnuts
1 cup raw sunflower seeds
1 Tbsp cold-pressed extra-virgin olive oil or unprocessed coconut oil
1 tsp Nama Shoyu
1 tsp chili powder

To make:
Soak the almonds, pecans, hazelnuts and sunflower seeds in pure water overnight. Rinse in the morning.
In a blender, add the olive or coconut oil, Nama Shoyu, chili powder and blend. Use this to coat the nuts. Dehydrate 8-10 hours or until dry.

Recipe by Brigitte Mars, www.brigittemars.com

Blond Ambition

Ingredients:
1½ cups hulled sesame seeds (unsoaked)
¾ cup unsweetened shredded coconut
½ cup raw tahini
¼ cup raw almond butter
½ - ¾ cup raw agave or raw honey
½ Tbsp psyllium powder (optional)

To make:
Combine tahini, almond butter, and agave (or honey) in a bowl. Add the rest of the ingredients and mix well. Spread the mixture into a 9 by 13 inch pan, smoothing with spatula.
Place in the refrigerator until firm. Cut into triangles or bars.

Recipe by Nadhirrah; email nadhirrah@care2.com

Kale chips
Serves 3

Ingredients:

1 head kale
4 Tbsp cold-pressed extra-virgin olive oil
1 Tbsp Nama shoyu
3 Tbsp spirulina
1 lemon, freshly squeezed juice of
1 pinch Celtic sea salt
2 cloves garlic or 1 Tbsp garlic powder

To make:

Rip or cut kale into bite size pieces and place them into a large mixing bowl. Add olive oil and mix until all the kale seems to be saturated. Add Nama shoyu and spirulina. Sprinkle lemon juice, salt, and minced garlic over the top.
Mix the contents of the bowl thoroughly.

To serve:

Option 1: Serve as is as a salad.
Option 2: For crunchy chips, tear the kale into large pieces before adding the rest of the ingredients, let marinate ½ hour, drain and dehydrate at 100 degrees overnight.
Option 3: Marinate slices of sweet onions in Nama shoyu overnight. Drain them and dehydrate the sliced onion with the kale chips and serve them together.

Recipe by Matthew Barraza; conan@inbox.com

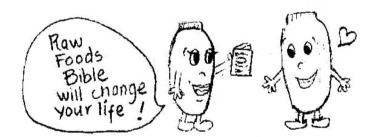

Red Beet Ravioli with Yellow Pepper Puree and Cashew Cheese

Serves 4–6

Ingredients Cashew Cheese:

2 cups raw cashews, soaked several hours
2½ Tbsp lemon juice, freshly squeezed
3 Tbsp nutritional yeast
1 tsp grated lemon zest
2 Tbsp minced scallion
2 Tbsp minced tarragon
1 Tbsp minced parsley
Unprocessed sea salt, to taste
Pure water (enough to make smooth)

To make Cashew Cheese:

Blend everything except scallion and herbs in a food processor (Cuisinart) with the S blade until smooth, adding small amounts of water if necessary. Place mixture into a bowl. Mix in minced herbs, add sea salt to taste.

Ingredients Yellow Pepper Puree:

3 yellow peppers (or try with red or orange peppers)
1 Tbsp lemon juice, freshly-squeezed
1 Tbsp white part of scallion
1 tsp unprocessed sea salt
1 Tbsp olive oil
½ cup pine nuts, soaked several hours
Note: if using red or orange peppers add a small pinch of ground turmeric.

To make Yellow Pepper Puree:

Puree in a high speed blender or Vita-Mix until smooth.

Ingredients for assembly:

Red beets, peeled and sliced thin on mandoline – stack the slices and cut into squares.
Pistachios, (preferably Sicilian) coarsely chopped
Tarragon, coarsely chopped or torn
Macadamia oil, cold pressed
Lemon juice, freshly-squeezed
Coarse sea salt and freshly ground black pepper

To assemble:

Pour macadamia oil into small dish – squeeze lemon into it. Dip each beet slice in oil/lemon. Place flat on plate. Sprinkle with sea salt. Add about 1 tsp of cashew cheese on each slice. Top with another beet slice, dipped in oil/lemon. Press down gently to secure. Sprinkle with sea salt. Spoon yellow pepper puree around it and sprinkle with pistachios, tarragon, and black pepper.

Recipe by Mathew of Pure Food and Wine, www.purefoodandwine.com

Breakfast

Sweet and Healthy Cereal
Serves 2

Ingredients:

3 Tbsp golden flax seeds

3 Tbsp brown flax seeds

6 sun-dried kalamata figs

¼ cup sun-dried raisins

¼ tsp cinnamon

½ cup pine nuts for cream (see recipe for Ricotta Cheese / Cream)

To make:

Soak figs overnight. Soak raisins from 15 mins. to overnight (save the liquid from the soaking).

Chop the figs into small pieces after soaking. In a coffee bean grinder or Vitamix, grind the dry flax seeds into meal.

Mix the flax meal and the liquid from the figs and raisins in a bowl (add liquid slowly, mixing with a fork each time you put more in so that the flax meal can fluff up because it tends to clump).

After the desired consistency is reached, add raisins, fig pieces and cinnamon, and then mix again.

Pour pine nut cream on top and serve! Yummy!!

Recipe by Katherine Narava Kaufman, www.simplylovingraw.com

Crunchy Buckwheat Granola
Serves up to 25

Ingredients:

4 pounds buckwheat, soaked for a few hours and rinsed

½ pound raw sunflower seeds, soaked 4-6 hours

½ pound sesame seeds, soaked 4-6 hours

½ pound pumpkin seeds, soaked 4-6 hours

½ pound flax seeds, soaked 4-6 hours

4 ounces shredded coconut

1½ Tbsp cinnamon

½ pound dried currants, not soaked

2 pounds honey dates, pitted and soaked for a few hours

To make:

Put dates in blender with enough water to form a paste.

Combine all ingredients and hand mix.

Spread evenly onto dehydrator trays covered with teflex or parchment paper and dehydrate at 105 degrees until crispy throughout (approximately 24 hours).

Note: Spread approximately 6 cups of the mixture on each Excaliber dehydrator tray.

Recipe by Cheri Soria.

Sunshine Cereal
Serves 2

Ingredients:

1 mango, or apple, or orange, peeled, remove seeds and cube

1 banana, sliced

1/4 cup sunflower seeds, soaked several hours, rinsed well and lightly chopped

1/4 cup almonds, soaked 8-12 hours, rinsed well and lightly chopped

1/4 cup buckwheaties (buckwheat groats soaked 8-12 hours and air-dried or dehydrated)

1/8 cup dried cranberries (unsweetened and unsulfured)

Orange Vanilla Mylk (see recipe in the Nut and Seed Milk section)

To make:

Place ingredients equally into 2 bowls. Add Orange-Vanilla Mylk for a nutritious and delicious way to add sunshine to your day!

Recipe by Ani Phyo, www.smartmonkeyfoods.com

Nature's Antioxidant Blast
Serves 2 or more

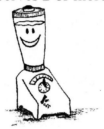

Ingredients:

¼ cup blueberries (frozen are OK for all berries)

¼ cup raspberries

¼ cup strawberries (organic only!)

¼ cup blackberries (omit if diverticula pockets are a problem)

¼ cup pitted cherries

1 ripe banana

1 Tbsp ground flax seeds

1 Tbsp shelled hemp seeds

1 Tbsp barley grass powder

1 tsp chlorella powder

1 Tbsp non-GMO lecithin granules

¼ tsp virgin (unprocessed) coconut oil (optional)

¼ tsp turmeric powder or a coin-sized slice of fresh turmeric

¼ tsp ginger powder or a coin size-sliced of fresh ginger, minced

1 dash cinnamon

1 dash cayenne powder (optional) or part of a fresh pepper

2–4 whole cloves or ¼ tsp clove powder

1–2 cups pure water

To make:

Place all ingredients in a blender and blend until smooth. Enjoy!

Recipe by Craig Sommers, www.rawfoodsbible.com

Victoria's Secret

Ingredients:
9 ounces of purified water
2 ripe bananas
1 apple, sliced
1½ Tbsp of chopped pitted dates
2 collard green leaves, torn into pieces
To make:
Place all ingredients in a blender and blend until smooth.
Recipe by Arnolds Way, www.arnoldsway.com

Eric's Breakfast Puree

Ingredients:
1 cucumber (peeled if not organic)
1 avocado
1 handful dark green leafy vegetable such as arugula or lacinato kale
freshly squeezed lime juice, to taste
To make:
Place all ingredients in a food processor and process with the S blade until smooth
Variations:
Sweeter version, add stevia, ginger or cinnamon/nutmeg to taste.
Saltier version: replace lime juice with unprocessed sea salt and pizza or Italian spice by Frontier Spices.
Recipe by Eric Prouty, www.quantumsnacks.com

Mixed Fruit Spread
Makes about 2 cups

Ingredients:
1 large apple
1 large pear
1 large ripe banana
12 strawberries
1 tsp freshly squeezed lemon juice
To make:
Peel, core and slice the apple and pear. Slice up the banana. Wash and remove the leaves from the strawberries. Place the apple and pear slices in a blender and blend on slow for a few seconds. Add the rest of the ingredients and blend again for a minute or so. Do not blend for too long or it will liquefy.
Recipe by Gloria Drnjevic, glovegan@yahoo.com

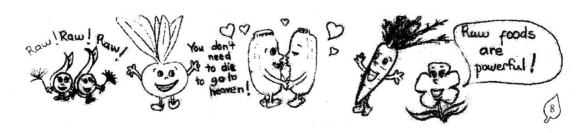

Yogurt

Preface to Yogurt Recipes

During the fermentation of traditional yogurt, a mixed culture of beneficial bacteria, including lactobacillus varieties, proliferate. Yogurt's acidity helps to inhibit the growth of bad bacteria, and its good bacteria aid in replenishing beneficial intestinal flora that are essential for vibrant health.

Good sterile technique is crucial when making yogurt. Since we're skipping the traditional step of boiling the milk to kill off unfriendly bacteria, and since the object here is to multiply good bacteria, we should be extra careful to keep everything as clean and sterile as possible. This is particularly important for the glass jars in which the yogurt incubates.

The starter that I use is called Jarro-Dophilus + FOS (dairy free powder). It is a high-potency probiotic with 6 types of bacteria and a total of 12 billion bacteria organisms per ¼ teaspoon. It produces a great tasting yogurt. Look for it at natural foods stores. Keep it refrigerated. Other probiotic powders with different bacteria combinations may produce different flavors and results, and different amounts will likely be needed. (If you use a low potency acidophilus, use more starter).

Lactobacillus (the healthy bacteria that makes yogurt) is killed above 130F, and does not thrive (but still grows) below 98F.

Thai Coconut Yogurt
Makes 1 quart

Ingredients:

¼ tsp Jarrow-Dophilus (Using less slows down the process, using more does not make a difference.)

1 quart Thai coconut cream (Thai Young Coconuts may be dipped in a chemical bath, including formaldehyde, to kill parasites in the husk. They are not organic.)

To Make Coconut Cream:

Use a small knife to cut off any patches of light brown inner shell that may still be stuck to the meat. Small amounts are not a problem. You can eat these cut-off pieces, but be careful of any fragments of hard outer shell that may have come off with the coconut meat. Put the cleaned coconut meat in a blender and blend it with some coconut water to obtain a smooth and creamy consistency. You can make it as thick or thin as you want by adjusting the amount of coconut water used (both thick and thin work fine).

To make Yogurt:

While the coconut cream is still in the blender, gently blend in the starter (because over-agitation before incubation may kill some of the bacteria and slow down the process).

Pour into a "sterile" jar to incubate. Place a chef's instant-read thermometer into the jar so that you can keep an eye on the temperature of the yogurt while it is incubating.

Incubating: The most frequently recommended incubation temperature for yogurt is 110F, with the most frequently cited acceptable range being 108F to 112F. Both high and low temperatures slow down culture growth and increase incubation time. I like a very tart yogurt, so I incubate the yogurt for about 18 hours. Incubate for a shorter period if you prefer a milder flavor. You may prefer the results after only 6 hours.

Here are a few incubating techniques:

Option 1. Electric Heating Pad:

Place an 8"x8"x2" deep glass baking dish on an electric heating pad and place 4 one-quart mason jars of yogurt mixture in it along with an instant read thermometer wedged between two of the jars with the readout dial hanging off of the edge of the baking dish. I then fill the baking dish with 130F water, which immediately drops to below 100F because the jars absorb the heat. I cover the jars with another upside-down 8"x8" glass baking dish and set the electric heating pad to high. The temperature of the water bath and the yogurt slowly rises to about 105F and stays at that temperature, a bit short of ideal, but it works. Using glass baking dishes keeps the yogurt constantly visible for monitoring. You could use a large covered pot instead. Placing everything into a covered box or ice chest may help by retaining more heat.

Option 2. Gas Oven Pilot Flame:

Many people use a gas oven with only the pilot flame lit. If this keeps the oven temperature too high, say at about 150F, they put the glass jars in a water bath in a large pot to keep the temperature in the right range [or leave the oven door ajar].

Option 3. Excalibur Dehydrator:

Place the jars into the dehydrator along with an instant-read thermometer so that you can keep an eye on the temperature in the dehydrator. Since Excalibur dehydrators run about 20F hotter than what you set them at, you will have to set the temperature dial at about 90F to get a temperature that fluctuates roughly between 108F and 112F.

Flavoring: (optional):

Once the desired tartness is reached, blend in sweetener (I use 1 packet of stevia powder) & fruit as desired and refrigerate immediately.

How long does it last? I don't know, this stuff is so delicious that no matter how much I make, it's all gone within one day.

Recipe by Mark Wisdom, www.rawwisdom.com

Acidophilus, Hazelnut, and Almond Yogurts

Ingredients:

1 tsp nondairy acidophilus powder (Jarrow-Dophilus by Jarrow, is a high-potency multi-strain product that I recommend).

1 quart living almond milk or hazelnut milk (see recipe in this section) or organic unsweetened soy milk (The ingredients should be soybeans and water, nothing else. Westsoy brand in aseptic containers works great.) Thick nut milk works better than watery; be sure to strain and discard the nut skins.

To make:

Pour the acidophilus powder into the milk of your choice and mix well. Use a sterile mason jar or any clean glass jar. Let stand at room temperature (warmer is better) for 24-48 hours or use one of the methods for incubation in the Thai Coconut Yogurt recipe. Be sure not to introduce any saliva into the yogurt with a used spoon or with your lips when tasting; it can ruin the culture. The milk will coagulate and separate. The soy yogurt can stay at room temperature for a few days after culturing but refrigerate the nut yogurts after culturing. The first batch is the starter for future batches; use a tablespoon of the thick part to inoculate the next batch. The friendly bacteria (acidophilus) will become specific to the medium (soy, almond or hazelnut) and grow better, achieving a creamier yogurt, with each batch.

This food is very beneficial to the intestines/digestive tract and the immune system!

Store-bought yogurt does not have live acidophilus cultures in it unless it says so.

They pasteurize it for longer shelf life, which kills the beneficial bacteria (acidophilus).

Recipe by Craig Sommers, www.rawfoodsbible.com

Nondairy Milks and Beverages

Almond, Brazil, Hazelnut, and Sunflower Milks

Ingredients:

Nuts or seeds of choice

Pure water

Sweetener of your choice, a soft date, raw agave, raw honey, or stevia

1 pinch of unprocessed sea salt

To make:

Place soaked almonds or hazelnuts (soak 12 hrs. and discard soak water) or sunflower seeds or Brazil nuts (soak 3 hrs. and discard soak water) in a blender, so that the nuts are even with the level of the uppermost part of the blades. Add pure water to just cover the nuts and blend until smooth. Add more water until desired consistency is reached. Sweeten to suit your taste buds with a soft date or two, raw agave, raw honey or a packet of stevia powder (if you use too much stevia, it will become bitter). Strain with cheesecloth or a nut milk bag. I use a paint strainer bag from the hardware store. Make only what you will use in one day. Refrigerate. These milks will go bad after about 24 hours although they will last longer if you are making yogurt with them.

Recipe by Craig Sommers, www.rawfoodsbible.com

Almond Strawberry Mylk
Serves 5 or more

Ingredients:

3 cups almonds, soaked overnight

7 cups coconut water (pure water will do if coconuts are not available)

2 cups strawberries

¼ cup raw carob powder

2 tsp mesquite powder (optional)

½ vanilla bean, scraped or ground or 2 tsp vanilla extract

½ tsp Himalayan salt (or Celtic sea salt)

To make:

In two batches, blend almonds and coconut water and strain through a nut bag (or paint strainer bag or nylon mesh). Pour mylk back into blender and blend with other ingredients until smooth and creamy. (Optional: Reserve pulp, dehydrate and grind into flour.)

Recipe by Tree Of Life Café.

Orange Vanilla Mylk
Yields about 4 cups

Ingredients:

½ cup pecans, soaked 6-8 hours and rinsed well

1 cup raw almonds, soaked 8-12 hours and rinsed well

1/3 cup pitted dates or a cored apple for a lower gycemic index

½ vanilla bean

1 orange, peeled and sliced

1 Tbsp virgin coconut oil

2-3 cups pure water

To make:

Place everything in a blender and blend. Delicious nutmylk in seconds!

Keeps for 3 days in the refrigerator.

Recipe by Ani Phyo, www.smartmonkeyfoods.com

Gimme Good Stuff Almond Milk

Ingredients:

1½ cups raw almonds (dry measure 1½ cups (8 oz), soaked measure 2½ cups (12 oz)

½ cup (5 oz) pitted dates

1½ Tbsp flax seeds

3 quarts pure water

To make:

Soak almonds in pure water for 8 hours and rinse thoroughly before making milk.

Blend all dry ingredients and 1 quart water until smooth.

For smooth milk (our favorite!) strain milk through a milk bag (see our website). If you don't have one, a clean nylon stocking or cotton pillowcase works fine too!

We use the pulp that remains in soups, breads or crackers.

You now have almond milk concentrate! Use it as is, or do what we do and dilute with 2 quarts more water. Use the milk fresh or freeze for later use. Place frozen jar into warm tap water to thaw. Shake well before serving; milk will separate as it sits.

Recipe by Good Stuff by Mom & Me, Raw, Vegan, Organic, Germinated, Gluten-free Good Foods! www.gimmegoodstuff.com

e-mail: info@gimmegoodstuff.com

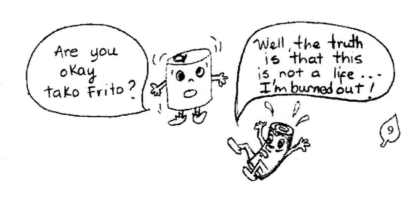

Hemp Seed Milk

Ingredients:

¼ cup shelled hempseeds (buy them in air-tight containers, not from bulk bins where they can be rancid)

1 liter pure water

1 pinch of unprocessed sea salt (optional)

1 soft date or 1 Tbsp raw honey or agave nectar or 1 packet stevia powder (do not add more stevia or it will produce a bitter taste), or sweetener of your choice

To make:

Place the hempseeds in a blender with just enough water to cover them and blend well. Add the rest of the ingredients and blend until smooth. Strain in a mesh strainer and drink! Refrigerate the remainder.

Optional: For a thicker, more omega-three-rich milk, soak ¼ cup flax seeds for 2 hours, rinse and blend with hemp seeds.

Recipe by Tenasi Rama.

Raw 'Soy' Milk

Ingredients:

1½ cups coconut water

½ cup raw rice bran

To make:

Mix it in the blender. Serve.

Recipe by Ito.

Raw Rice Dream

Ingredients:

1½ cups pure water

½ cup raw rice bran

1 Tbsp raw agave

To make:

Mix it in a blender. Serve.

Variations:

Add raw carob powder, cacao, durian, or whatever else your heart desires.

Recipe by Ito.

Golden Milk
Yields 3 cups

Ingredients:

2 cups pure water

½ cup pine nuts

1 Tbsp unrefined coconut oil

1/8th tsp cinnamon

1/8th tsp stevia powder or sweetener of choice

1 Tbsp turmeric powder or diced fresh root

1 Tbsp chopped fresh ginger root (optional)

1 pinch cayenne powder (optional)

2 Tbsp goji berries (optional)
1/8th tsp unprocessed sea salt (optional)
To make:
Place all ingredients in a blender and blend until smooth. If using a weak blender and solid coconut oil, liquefy oil first by placing the jar in warm water until it melts.

    Recipe by Craig Sommers, adapted from Yogi Bhajan's cooked golden milk recipe www.rawfoodsbible.com

Lemonade Refresher
Yields 1 blender full

Ingredients:
2 lemons, freshly-squeezed juice of
½ lemon rind (organic only)
1 pinch unprocessed sea salt
1 tsp green leaf stevia powder
1 liter of pure water (as needed to fill blender)

To make:
Blend to desired frothiness and enjoy chilled or at room temperature.

    Recipe by Shakti Parvati, www.shaktiandthebluelotus.com

Lemon Melon Cooler
Yields 1 blender full

Ingredients:
3 lbs or ½ small watermelon
1 lemon, freshly squeezed juice of
½ tsp unprocessed sea salt
1 tsp white stevia powder
2 cups pure water (mix with ice if desired)
1 inch piece of ginger, diced

To make:
Place all ingredients into a blender and blend on high. Enjoy!

    Recipe by Shakti Parvati, www.shaktiandthebluelotus.com

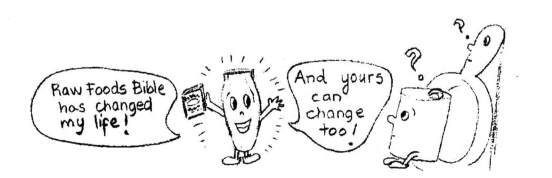

Rejuvelac

Rejuvelac is a beverage full of enzymes, friendly lactic acid bacteria (lactobacilli), aspergillus oryzae, vitamins B, E, K, proteins in the form of amino acids, carbohydrates (already broken down into the simple sugars, dextines and saccharines) and minerals. Besides being a beverage, Rejuvelac can also be used to ferment seed cheeses and loaves and to keep energy soups from oxidizing so they will last the whole day. There are two methods to make Rejuvelac. The first method is an adapted version for those new to sprouting and the second is the Ann Wigmore Version.

Ingredients:

1 cup soft white wheat berries

¼ cup rye berries (optional)

pure water

To make, method 1: Soak berries overnight in 3 cups filtered or distilled water. Drain and rinse. Replace filtered water. Soak overnight again and up to 2 - 3 days. It is finished when it has a slightly lemony flavor. Strain the rejuvelac into another container and refrigerate. You can keep the berries and dehydrate them for a breakfast cereal (add nuts, raisins and apples) or meal (add onions, ginger, garlic and vegetables) or make two more batches of rejuvelac. Just refill the original jar with water and allow fermenting again. Usually the rejuvelac is ready much sooner the second and third time around.

To make, method 2: Soak berries 6 - 8 hours (to germinate) in a thoroughly scrubbed clean jar with filtered or distilled water. Cover the mouth of the jar with a piece of mesh and a heavy rubber band to serve as a sieve. (Use fiberglass window screening.) DRAIN, do not rinse and let sprout for 2 days. Turn the jar upside down and lean it at an angle to allow complete drainage. Keep it out of direct sunlight. Rinse and drain 2 - 3 times daily for the next two days by filling the jar with water, agitating and pouring the water out again at least 3 times in succession.

The idea is to keep the berries moist and clean, but continually exposed to air. The berries will begin to sprout tails. Continue this sprouting process until the tails are approximately equal in length to the berries. Rinse the sprouts thoroughly before proceeding to the Fermentation Process.

NOW POUR WATER over sprouted wheat seeds. Use about 3 times the amount of water as there are seeds. (The water is now absorbing nutrients from the sprouts)

COVER JAR with wire mesh or cheese cloth and let stand at room temperature for approximately 48 hours (time will vary with room temperature). Stir and taste once each day until the water acquires a slightly sour taste. When the water tastes sour (somewhat reminiscent of unsweetened lemonade/cheese/sauerkraut) it is ready to use.

A white surface film is acceptable and desirable. Pour off liquid into another container and store in refrigerator to retard the fermentation process. It will keep for several days in the refrigerator so long as the taste/aroma/appearance remains the same.

Then use leftover wheat seeds and soak again another 24 hours (the second batch will be ready more quickly than the first batch) for two more times to make two more batches of rejuvelac. Discard or compost wheat seeds when you are done.

IF YOUR REJUVELAC HAS A FUNKY SMELL dump it out and start again. Wheat berries are inexpensive and it may take you a couple of times before you get it correct. The taste is supposed to be like unsweetened tart lemonade.

Recipes by Deva Khalsa, www.thecleanse.com

Sangria O'live Punch
Serves 6

Ingredients:

3 cups grapes (red or white)

2/3 cup lemon juice, freshly squeezed

2/3 cup lime juice, freshly squeezed

1 cup orange juice, freshly squeezed

1 cup apple juice, freshly juiced

1 handful of fresh mint leaves

1 orange, 6 thin slices for garnish and the remainder peeled and diced

1 apple, 6 thin slices for garnish and the remainder diced

1 handful of fresh and/or frozen grapes to garnish punch bowl & keep chilled

Optional: 2 Tbsp agave nectar or 3 pitted dates or 3 Tbsp raw honey or to taste or 1 cup freshly-squeezed pineapple juice

To make:

1 Process the 3 cups of grapes and lemon juice in a blender until smooth. Strain out the seeds.

2 Leave 6 mint leaves for garnishing and mash the rest into a large glass bowl (or a punch bowl) using the back of a spoon to press out the mint oils.

3 Pour the mixture into the glass bowl and add the other juices and diced fruit. Stir well.

4 Refrigerate until cold.

To Serve:

When ready to serve, float the handful of grapes in the punch bowl. Garnish top of punch bowl with slices of the apple and orange and whole mint leaves. Serve with a slice of orange or apple on the rim of each glass and with fresh diced fruit.

Keeps for 2-3 days in the refrigerator.

Recipe by Kimberly Mac, www.thenakedvegan.com

Raw Chai
Serves 4

Ingredients:

1 cup raw cashews

3 cups pure water or coconut water

2 Tbsp unprocessed coconut oil

2 tsp cardamom powder

1 tsp clove powder

1 pinch Celtic sea salt

2 inch piece of fresh ginger root, peeled and grated

To make:

In a high speed blender, add all ingredients and blend until smooth.

Recipe by Tone Anthony of Norway, owner of *Art of Raw Food*.

Pâtés, Spreads, and Nondairy Cheeses

Omega Three Pâté
Serves 2-4

Ingredients:

1½ cups walnut halves soaked from 4-6 hours and rinsed (taste first to make sure the nuts are not rancid)
1 cup chopped asparagus
1 medium tomato (Roma tomato recommended)
½ cup chopped parsley (stems also)
2 cloves garlic or 1 tsp asafetida powder (garlic substitute)
4 tsp fresh-squeezed lemon juice
2 Tbsp unpasteurized mellow white miso

To make:

Place all ingredients in a food processor and process until smooth.
Recipe by Craig Sommers, www.rawfoodsbible.com

Jai To The Most High Sunflower Seed Dip
Serves 2-3

15 minutes + soaking time

Ingredients:

1 cup sunflower seeds, soaked at least 3 hours
¼ cup lemon juice, freshly squeezed
½ cup pure water
2 medium sun-dried tomatoes, soaked in warm water for 20 minutes
2 Tbsp Red bell pepper, diced
1 Tbsp Green onion, diced
1 Tbsp Olives, sliced thin
2 tsp basil, minced
2 tsp Italian parsley, minced
1 tsp apple cider vinegar, raw
1 tsp Nama shoyu, or to taste
½ tsp garlic, minced (optional)
¼ tsp oregano, fresh minced
¼ tsp unprocessed sea salt, or to taste
¼ tsp black pepper, ground to taste

To make:

1. Drain the sun-dried tomatoes and chop them into small pieces. Place them into a large mixing bowl.
2. Place soaked and drained sunflower seeds, lemon juice, water and garlic in food processor and process until smooth.
3. Place all ingredients in the large bowl and mix well. For best results allow to sit for a few hours before serving.

Serving suggestions:
Serve as a stuffing in a large tomato or red bell pepper as the main component of a large mixed green salad.
It can also be served as a spread for sandwiches or in live nori rolls.

Recipe reprinted from *Vegan World Fusion Cuisine* www.veganfusion.com, the cookbook and 'wisdom work' from the chefs of the Blossoming Lotus Restaurant on Kauai, HI. www.blossominglotus.com

Southwest Style Pâté
Serves 6-8

Ingredients:
1 cup pecans or sunflower seeds (soaked for a few hours first)
½ cup chopped carrots
½ cup chopped celery
½ cup chopped broccoli
¼ cup chopped onion
1 Tbsp minced garlic
1 Tbsp nori flakes
½ Tbsp grated ginger
1 tsp sea salt (or 1 Tbsp chickpea miso)
1 tsp cumin
Add some jalapeno, habanero or other chili powder, to give it a kick! (optional)
¼ cup freshly-squeezed orange juice
2 Tbsp apple cider vinegar
1 Tbsp flax oil

To make:
Place all ingredients except the last three in a food processor and process until smooth. Then add the last three ingredients while the processor is running, and process a little more.

Recipe by Bruce Horowitz; email chef_sprout2001@yahoo.com

Beet Pâté
Serves 4-6

Ingredients:
2 medium-sized beets
1 apple
2 inches of horseradish root
1 cup parsley, chopped
½ lemon, freshly-squeezed juice of
1 tsp raw apple cider vinegar
2 Tbsp Nama shoyu or unprocessed sea salt to taste
2 tsp psyllium husk powder

To make:
Cut the horseradish into small pieces and process in a food processor with the S blade until smooth. Shred the beets and apple with a mandolin or with a food processor using the shredding disc. Set aside some shredded apples and beets for decorating the top of the pâté when finished.
Place all ingredients in the food processor and process using the S blade until a smooth consistency is reached.

Serving suggestions:
Place a scoop of pâté on a lettuce leaf or fill a Belgium endive leaf like a boat and garnish.

This is Ursula's grandmother's recipe for springtime cleansing. She says to pay attention because it is a real blood and colon cleanser!

Recipe by Ursula Horaitis, www.goodmoodfood.com

Down-to-the-Roots Pâté
Serves 2-4

Ingredients:
1 large sweet potato or yam (peeled if not organic)
1 small beet (peeled if not organic)
1 small carrot (peeled if not organic)
1 clove of garlic or ½ tsp asafetida powder
1 or 2 slices of onion or more to taste
1 Tbsp freshly ground ginger (or less if you don't like ginger)
1 tsp turmeric powder or 1 Tbsp fresh root
½ tsp cumin
½ tsp coriander
½ - 1 tsp unprocessed sea salt (to taste)
1 pinch of black pepper (fresh ground)
3 Tbsp cold-pressed, extra-virgin olive oil

To make:
Chop and then process all the ingredients in a food processor using the S blade.

Suggested use:
Serve as burrito filling wrapped in your favorite leaves and topped with such delights as sprouts, avocado, and scallions, use it for dipping carrot and celery sticks or spread onto Essene bread.

Recipe by Guru Beant Kamke.

Asian Pâté
Serves 6-8

Ingredients:

1 cup of raw almonds soaked for 24 hrs (to germinate)
2 cups of sunflower seeds soaked for 6 hrs (or overnight) and sprouted for 1-2 days
¼ cup lemon juice, freshly-squeezed
¾ cup fresh onion, chopped
2 garlic cloves
1½ cups celery
¾ cup parsley
1½ cups red bell pepper
½ cup Nama Shoyu [or ¼ cup for a less salty taste]
½ cup dulse flakes
2 Tbsp kelp granules

To make:

In a food processor, process the almonds, sunflower seeds, ¼ cup of fresh lemon juice, ¾ cup of fresh onion, and 2 garlic cloves. Run the processor until the ingredients become a paste; you may need to stop the processor several times and work the mixture away from the sides of the processor bowl. Once done, put the resulting paste into a mixing bowl. Then mince and mix in the remaining ingredients:

This paté is great on its own, in a nori roll with lots of fresh vegetables and daikon sprouts, as a salad topping, or whatever your imagination will come up with!

Recipe by Elizabeth Michael.

Pumpkin Seed Pâté
Serves 6

Ingredients:

1 pound raw pumpkin seeds (before soaking)
4 cloves garlic, medium-sized

To make:

Soak the pumpkin seeds in pure water, in a warm place, for 16 to 24 hours.
Drain and rinse the seeds. Process the soaked seeds and garlic in a food processor, using the S blade, or a high speed blender such as a Vitamix (if using a blender add a small amount of water so it blends easier).

To Serve:

Spread it on top of thinly sliced vegetables such as zucchini or inside of celery.

Recipe by Shui Lau Neric.

Mock Salmon Pâté
Makes 4 cups

Ingredients:

2 cups soaked almonds (soak overnight)
2 medium carrots
¼ cup carrot juice (about 1½ large carrots)
3 Tbsp freshly squeezed lemon juice or more to taste (about 1 lemon)
1½ ribs finely diced celery
4 scallions finely chopped
2 tsp kelp powder
1 Tbsp Nama Shoyu or ½ tsp Celtic sea salt (or more)
[I also add 2 Tbsp of dulse flakes for extra flavor]

To make:

Put almonds, carrots, carrot juice, lemon juice and kelp powder through a food processor using the S blade, until creamy. Add Nama Shoyu or salt and process a little more. Mix the chopped scallions and diced celery with the contents of the food processor by hand in a bowl.

To serve:

Spread onto sliced cucumber or flax crackers or place in the middle of a green salad.

Recipe by Elaina Love, www.purejoyivingfoods.com

Lou-ney Tuna
Serves 4

Ingredients:

2 cups almonds soaked 24 hours
3-4 ribs celery cut into bite size pieces
4-5 carrots cut into bite-sized pieces
1 cup fresh parsley, chopped
2 tsp kelp powder
¼ cup dulse flakes
1 tsp Celtic sea salt
2 Tbsp freshly squeezed lemon juice

To make:

Place all ingredients in a large bowl and stir. Run the mixture through a Champion Juicer or a food processor using the S blade.

Serving suggestions:

Add chopped red onion, green onion, chopped celery or shredded carrot to pate (by hand mixing).

Place pate inside of collard greens or romaine leaves or on top of cucumber slices, or inside of red bell pepper. Top with sliced cherry tomatoes and avocado.

Recipe by Elaina Love, www.purejoyivingfoods.com

Powerful Pesto
Makes approximately 2 cups

Ingredients:

1 cup pine nuts or soaked pecans
1/3 cup walnuts (soaked for 3 hours and rinsed)
1/2 cup cold-pressed extra-virgin olive oil
1/4 cup nutritional yeast (not a raw product)
2 cups fresh basil
1-2 cloves of garlic
1/2 tsp fresh rosemary or ¼ tsp dry rosemary
1/2 tsp fresh sage or ¼ tsp dry sage
1/2 tsp unprocessed sea salt

To make:

Process everything in a food processor using the S blade until creamy. Pesto can be stored in a refrigerator for several weeks if a layer of olive oil is poured on top of the pesto.

Recipe by Christina Ott, www.barefootbuiulder.com

No Bean Hummus

Ingredients:

2 zucchinis, diced
2 lemons, either whole peeled or freshly-juiced
6-8 cloves of garlic
½ cup cold-pressed extra-virgin olive oil
½ cup raw, unsalted tahini
1 cup parsley, chopped
2-4 Tbsp Nama shoyu or unprocessed sea salt to taste

To make:

Place all ingredients except the tahini in a blender and mix to a thick creamy consistency. Then add the tahini and mix again.

Recipe by Ursula Horaitis, www.goodmoodfood.com

Living Laughing Creamy Hummus
Serves 4-6

Ingredients:

2 cups sprouted chickpeas
½ cup extra-virgin, cold-pressed olive oil
1 tsp flax oil (optional)
4 cloves raw garlic or 2 tsp asafetida powder
1 lemon, juice of
1 tsp unprocessed sea salt
1 Tbsp unpasteurized mellow white miso
1 Tbsp raw tahini
2½ Tbsp raw macadamia or raw cashew butter
3 Tbsp *water* from soaked kalamata figs (not the figs themselves). Let figs soak 6-8 hrs.

To make:

Place all of the ingredients into a high-quality food processor, blender or Vitamix. Blend until smooth. **For optimum flavor,** store in refrigerator for 24 hrs. before eating.

Suggested uses:

Spread into celery ribs, bok choy and red pepper quarters.
Recipe by Craig Sommers, www.rawfoodsbible.com

Salmon Spread
Serves 6

Ingredients:

1 cup raw cashews
1 cup almonds, soaked overnight and rinsed
1 cup sunflower seeds, soaked overnight and rinsed
1 rib celery
½ medium-sized red bell pepper
2 scallions
½ tsp unprocessed sea salt
1/8 tsp white pepper
2 tsp nori flakes or granules
1 tsp dulse flakes or granules
1 tsp garlic, minced
2 Tbsp freshly squeezed lemon juice
2 Tbsp cold-pressed extra-virgin olive oil
1½ tsp Nama shoyu

To make:

Place cashews, salt, pepper, nori, dulse, garlic, lemon juice, olive oil, Nama shoyu, and bell pepper in a food processor. Run on high until smooth.

Place remaining ingredients in the food processor. Run on high until semi-smooth and still a bit grainy. For best flavor, refrigerate several hours before serving.
Recipe by Brad Wolff, Vegan Food Scientist/Product Developer;
email veganfoods@yahoo.com

Ricotta Cheese/Cream

Ingredients:

1 cup pine nuts

1 cup water

dash of unprocessed sea salt (optional)

To make:

Process nuts and water in a blender. Pour contents of blender into a sprouting bag (a paint strainer bag works well and is available at a hardware store) and squeeze out the liquid (if nothing is left in the bag you processed the nuts too long). The liquid is pine nut cream and is excellent on breakfast cereal. The ricotta cheese is what is left in the bag. Add salt if desired.

Recipe by Craig Sommers, www.rawfoodsbible.com

Spreadable, Delectable Cheese

Ingredients:

2 cups raw macadamia nuts (check for freshness)

1 cup pine nuts

1 lemon, juice of

1 tsp unprocessed sea salt (or less if salt is not desired)

To make:

Place the nuts, salt and the juice of the lemon in a high-quality food processor, or Vitamix (tamper needed for Vitamix). Blend until smooth. Eat very soon and refrigerate any leftovers in a sealed container.

Variations:

Add a small amount of turmeric powder for yellow cheese or add any spices desired.

(I have used 2 cups pine and one cup macadamia with excellent results.)

Dehydrate for hard cheese!

Keeps in refrigerator for at least two weeks.

Recipe by Jackie Graff, www.sproutcafe.com

Live "Sour Cream"
Serves 4

Ingredients:

2 cups raw cashews or macadamias (soak nuts for a few hours before using)

½ cup lemon juice, freshly squeezed

½ tsp unprocessed sea salt

To make:

Using the S blade, process all ingredients in a food processor. If using a blender instead of a food processor, add ¼ cup of pure water.

Recipe by Amy Rachelle, www.amyrachelle.com

Cheddar Cheese Slices

Yields 2 trays in an Excalibur dehydrator

Ingredients:

3 cups hulled sesame seeds (soaking optional)

1 - 2 cups pure water

1 cup red bell pepper, chopped

1/4 cup freshly squeezed orange juice (the sweeter the orange the better)

1/8 cup freshly squeezed lemon juice

1 Tbsp fresh garlic, minced

1 Tbsp fresh turmeric, peeled and minced or 1-2 tsp turmeric powder

1 Tbsp flax oil

1 Tbsp Celtic sea salt (it needs the full 1 Tbsp)

1 Tbsp chopped onion

1/2 tsp fresh ginger, peeled and minced

Hot chili to taste (optional)

1/2 tsp ground white pepper (optional)

1/2 tsp coriander (optional)

To make:

In a food processor with the S blade, blend until creamy (start with one cup water, it may not need both cups). The mix will taste slightly bitter, but dehydration should cause the orange juice to sweeten it. It is an option to add extra sweetener at this time.

Spread 1/8-inch thick onto Teflex sheets and dehydrate until chewy.

This recipe needs longer food processing time and dehydration time than most.

Recipe by Bruce Horowitz; email: chef_sprout2001@yahoo.com

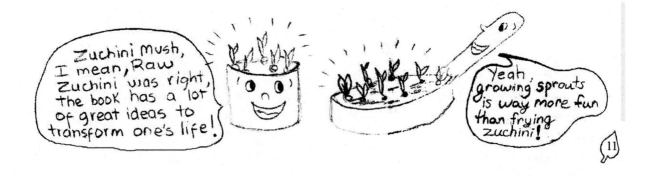

Pizza Crust, Sprouted Bread, and Crackers

Pizza Parlor Crust
Makes 2 Crusts

Ingredients:

1½ cups almonds (soaked 12 hours)

1 apple (deseeded and quartered)

¼ cup extra-virgin, cold-pressed olive oil

1 Tbsp Celtic sea salt

1½ Tbsp Italian seasoning (Frontier Herbs makes an organic one)

1¼ cups flax seeds (ground into meal)

1/3 cup pure water

To make:

In a food processor, using the S-blade, process the almonds on the highest setting. Add water, oil, salt and apple. Blend for 1 minute. Add herbs and then slowly pour in flax meal while machine is on. Mixture will begin to clump together. Continue to blend until mixture resembles a ball of dough. Section dough into 2 balls (more for smaller crusts). Place one ball on teflex (or onto parchment paper) and use wet fingers to spread dough around into a pizza-shaped circle. Dough should be ¼ inch thin. Form crust by folding edges over.

Dehydrate for 12 hours at 99 degrees (flip over after a few hours and remove Teflex sheet or parchment paper).

To make pizza, top with marinara (see recipe in Entrée section), macadamia-pine nut cheese (see recipe in Cheese section) and toppings (onions, red peppers, olives…).

Recipe by Karen Parker.

Italian Essene Bread / Breadsticks
Fills about 4 trays in a dehydrator (depending on thickness)

Ingredients:

5 cups sprouted kamut berries

4 cups sprouted spelt berries

2½ cups sprouted sunflower seeds

½ cup soaked pumpkin seeds (soak for a few hours)

½ sweet onion chopped finely

½ cup onion sprouts or any other sprouts (alfalfa, radish, clover…)

¼ cup fresh basil leaves finely chopped

2 Tbsp Italian seasoning (Frontier makes an organic one)

2 tsp unprocessed sea salt

1 Tbsp kelp powder

To make:

Place all ingredients in a large mixing bowl and spoon-mix very well. Processing the mixture is not easy unless the correct machine is used because the gluten in the grains clogs most machines and can burn out the motor. Process small amounts at a time if using a food processor or a Vitamix. With this method, check to be sure that all grains have been crushed; if just one is left uncrushed, it will be a hard piece in the finished bread that can be unpleasant to eat. The easiest way to process the mix into dough is with a corkscrew type of food processor such as the Omega 8001 or 8002 or 8003 juicer using the blank plate instead of the screen. I have used an old hand-crank meat grinder with great success for years!

Spread the batter thin on dehydrator trays lined with parchment paper using a spatula **or** if using the Omega 8001 or 8002 or 803 juicer, the processed dough comes out perfectly for bread sticks (form into pretzels or any fun shape)!

Dehydrate at 99 degrees for at least 12 hours or until dry. Dehydration time depends on many factors: the relative humidity (the higher the longer it takes), the ambient temperature and the thickness of the bread. I prefer to "cook" my bread in the sun when possible. For years I have prepared Essene bread in my camper and "cooked" it on the dashboard with the sun coming through the windshield. In New Mexico where the humidity is 20-30% and the elevation is 5000 feet above sea level, the bread is ready in a few hours. In the New England area, the same bread will take 2 days and acquires a fermented taste!

Flip the bread over when it becomes dry enough to do so.

Store the bread in a sealed container or zip-lock bag and refrigerate for optimum taste and nutrient retention. Essene bread is considered to be a fermented food by some and will continue to ferment if not fully dry and left out at room temperature. When fully dry, the bread can stay at room temperature for months.

Of all the grains, I have found that Kamut is the best tasting, least likely to mold, and easiest to process (because of its softness).

I encourage you to experiment with different spices and herbs. Endless recipes wait to be discovered!

Recipe by Craig Sommers (idea taken from the *Essene Gospel of Peace*).

EZ Essene Bread

Ingredients:
1 cup sprouted kamut berries (or wheat berries or spelt berries)
Spice as desired or not at all (refer to the Italian Essene bread recipe for ideas).
To Make:
Follow directions in the Italian Essene Bread recipe.
Recipe by Craig Sommers, www.rawfoodsbible.com

Black Sesame Crackers

Ingredients:
2 cups black sesame seeds
2 cups ripe bananas
1 tsp vanilla extract
To make:
Soak black sesame seeds in pure water for approximately 24 hours. Drain and rinse the seeds. Give the seeds about 24 hours to sprout by rinsing them a few times per day and keeping them well drained.

In a food processor using the S blade, process all the ingredients until mixed well.

Spread the mix thinly on non-bleached parchment paper or teflex dehydrator sheets. Dehydrate at 100 degrees for at least 8 hours (they may need more time depending on individual conditions) and then flip them over. Continue to dehydrate until they are very dry and crisp. Store in an airtight container, preferably in a cool place.

Recipe by Tone Anthony, owner of *Art of Raw Food.*

Quantum Health Crackers

Free yourself! Gluten Free, Grain Free, Yeast Free, Sugar Free!

Yield: 50-60 ounces, serving size: 1-2 ounces

Ingredients:

8 cups raw sunflower seeds
2 cups dry flax seeds
1 Tbsp minced garlic
2½ Tbsp Real Salt
2 Tbsp curry powder
3 Tbsp coriander
1 bunch kale
1 bunch celery
1 small head broccoli
1 head cabbage
1 onion
1 zucchini
1 lb. carrots
3¼ cups pure water

To make:

A. Soak sunflower seeds for four hours. Drain and puree in food processor (smooth puree not required). Set aside.

B. Make flour with flax seeds in blender (in ½ cup portions) or coffee grinder. Set aside.

C. Mix spices and salt in separate cup

C. Food process kale into 1/2" pieces, and add to large bowl.

D. Food process remaining vegetables into puree, Add to large bowl with sunflower seeds and seasonings and mix.

E. Add water to flax seed flour. Immediately whisk smooth and quickly transfer to vegetable puree. Mix thoroughly.

F. Spread smoothly onto Teflex sheets. Dehydrate at 140 degrees for 4 hours, flip crackers and peel off Teflex sheets, then reduce heat to 110-115 degrees. Make creases in crackers for easy breaking later. Continue dehydrating until crisp (approx 2 to 3 days, depending on the humidity of your house).

Variations:

For garlic lovers, replace curry and coriander with 2 Tbsp extra garlic and 2 tsp black pepper.

Notes:

This recipe should fill up a 9 tray Excalibur dehydrator.

As soon as veggies are pureed they become active, so work as fast as possible to get them into the dehydrator. Waiting too long results in fermentation of the mixture.

140 degrees in the beginning will not kill enzymes, because evaporation is a cooling process.

This is designed as a pH balancing grain replacement snack. This is a concentrated raw food, so eat with salsa, guacamole or Eric's Breakfast Puree (located in the Breakfast section).

Store in air tight containers. Will keep for 1-2 months If stored in a cool place.

Recipe by Eric Prouty, www.quantumsnacks.com

Flax Crackers, Pizza Flavored

Ingredients:

1 cup flax seeds (either brown, gold or a mix of both!)
1½ cups pure water
1 Tbsp Italian seasoning
1 tsp unprocessed sea salt (optional)

To make:

Soak the flax seeds in water for at least 4 hours, but not more than 8. After soaking, mix the gelatinous seeds (pour off extra water) with the spices (or spices of your choice).

Spread the mixture out on dehydrator trays lined with parchment paper or tray liner of choice. The thickness that works best is between 1/8- and 1/4-inch thick.

Dehydrate at 100 degrees Fahrenheit for about 24 hours or until crispy. I recommend flipping the crackers over when they become dry enough to do so.

Refrigerate after removing from dehydrator.

Recipe by Craig Sommers, www.rawfoodsbible.com

Russian Rye Crisps
Yields 4 trays

Ingredients:

5 cups sprouted rye
2 cups chopped red onion
2 cups chopped green cabbage
3 Tbsp kelp powder
4 Tbsp dulse flakes
3½ cups pure water

Toppings: (optional)

Dulse flakes
Caraway seed
Finely chopped red onion

To make:

In a blender, combine all ingredients except the toppings. Blend well until a thick batter is achieved. Pour onto a dehydrator tray using a Teflex sheet or unbleached parchment paper beneath.

Draw lines in the spread batter to form a pattern for separating the finished crackers. Sprinkle on desired toppings.

Dehydrate at 105 degrees overnight. Flip and dehydrate until completely crisp. Store in an airtight container or bag when completely dry.

Recipe by Kelly Serbonich, www.13ks.wholefoodfarmacy.com

Onion Flat Bread with Nut Cream Topping

Ingredients for bread:

2 cups sunflower seeds, soaked 3 hours and rinsed

2 cups almonds, soaked overnight and rinsed (they may also be dehydrated after soaking)

1 cup buckwheat groats, soaked for 1 hour and rinsed (dehydrating is optional)

1 lemon, freshly-squeezed juice of

3 Tbsp Nama Shoyu or a dash of unprocessed sea salt

Ingredients for nut cream:

1 cup raw cashews or raw macadamia nuts

1 lemon, freshly-squeezed juice of

1 tsp mustard (see recipe in Condiment section)

3 Tbsp Nama Shoyu or a dash of unprocessed sea salt or Herbamare

¼ cup cold-pressed extra-virgin olive oil

2 cups pure water

1 white onion, diced and marinated from 2 hours to overnight in a 50 / 50 mixture of Nama shoyu and pure water. (The strong essential oils are no longer present after marinating the onion and all that is left is a mild enjoyable flavor.)

Ingredients for decoration:

1 bunch parsley, chopped

To make bread:

Using a food processor with the S blade, process all the bread ingredients into dough. Press the dough into flat, square or round, thin (1/5 inch) patties using two plastic sheets (teflex dehydrator sheets work well.) Dehydrate (without teflex sheet) for about 8 hours.

To make cream:

Blend all ingredients except the onion and its marinade in a blender to achieve a creamy consistency and then place into a bowl. Drain onions well by squeezing the marinade out with your hands. Then add the onions to the cream and mix them in with a spoon.

To serve:

Spread the nut cream onto the dehydrated flat bread, decorate with parsley and serve.

This type of onion flatbread comes from Germany and France where it has been traditionally baked in a wood-fired oven.

Recipe by Ursula Horaitis, www.goodmoodfood.com

Igor's Crackers
Makes about 16 crackers

Ingredients:

3 ribs celery

1 large onion

2 tomatoes

2 cups flaxseed

4 cloves of garlic

1 tsp Celtic salt

1 tsp caraway seed

1 tsp coriander seed

1 cup pure water

To make:
Grind 2 cups flaxseed in a coffee bean grinder or dry Vitamix.

In a high-speed blender or Vitamix, blend the rest of the ingredients (excluding the flax meal). Add the flax meal to the mix and blend again until a slippery flax gel is formed (the mix should not be dry). Place the mix in a bowl, covered with cheesecloth or a towel and let it sit overnight at room temperature to ferment slightly. If a more sour taste is desired, ferment 2 – 3 days. Use a spatula to spread onto nonstick dehydrator sheets. Divide into squares of desired size. For soft crackers, dehydrate 16 hours, then flip and dehydrate for 4 more hours. For crispy crackers, dehydrate until crispy. Keep crackers refrigerated.

Recipe by The Raw Family, www.rawfamily.com

<u>Blueberry Hemp Lembas</u>

(These are the magical breads that the elves gave Frodo to nourish him on his journey in the Lord of the Rings.)

Ingredients:
1½ cups hulled hemp seeds
1 cup sprouted buckwheat
1 cup sprouted quinoa
1 cup soaked or sprouted sunflower seeds
¾ cup soaked pumpkin seeds
¾ cup soaked sesame seeds (hulled)
¾ cup soaked flax seeds
1 cup shredded coconut (sugar free)
2 cups pitted dates
2 cups fresh or frozen blueberries

To make:
Soak all the ingredients that require soaking for about 3 hours.

Using a food processor with the S blade, process a third of the buckwheat, quinoa and sunflower seeds and all of the dates to create a paste. Add the rest of the ingredients, except the blueberries, to the paste and hand mix. Stir clockwise 13 strokes, then counterclockwise 13 strokes, and repeat while imbuing the lembas with the power to nourish, sustain and liberate all who eat them. Use more or less shredded coconut to make mixture sticky. Spoon onto dehydrator sheets, traditionally in triangles, and press three blueberries on top of each lemba. Dehydrate until almost dry, or very dry for longer journeys.

Recipe by Tenasi Rama.

Entrées

Linguini Parody with White Truffle Cream
Serves 6

Ingredients:

1 ounce dried porcini mushrooms

1 cup water

8 medium zucchini, cut into long strips

2 tsp solar-dried, natural sea salt

Ingredients for sauce:

½ cup pine nuts, soaked 2 hours

½ cup cashews, soaked 2 hours

2 tsp white truffle oil

2 Tbsp freshly squeezed lemon juice

1 Tbsp fresh dill

1 Tbsp Nama Shoyu

1 Tbsp agave nectar

¼ tsp white pepper

Ingredients (other):

1 Tbsp dulse flakes

1 Tbsp kelp powder

¼ cup kombu, soaked 20 minutes and finely diced

1 cup Roma tomatoes, finely julienned

½ cup red onion, finely julienned

½ cup yellow bell pepper, finely julienned

¼ cup capers

¼ cup minced parsley, for garnish

fresh ground pepper, to taste

To make:

1. Combine dried porcini mushrooms with water to allow them to soften for 1 hour.

2. While the mushrooms are soaking, cut the zucchini into long thin strips resembling linguini (a Spirooli is perfect for this application). Sprinkle the salt on the zucchini noodles, toss well several times, and set aside.

3. After one hour, drain the mushrooms, reserving the water for use in the sauce. Dice the mushrooms and set aside.

4. Combine the ingredients for the sauce in a blender adding a small amount of the mushroom soaking water, as needed, to make a very thick creamy sauce.

5. Drain the zucchini noodles thoroughly (the salt will have drawn out some water), gently squeezing the noodles to remove more liquid, and then toss with the sauce and other remaining ingredients.

6. Garnish with minced parsley and a sprinkle of fresh ground pepper.

Recipe by Cherie Soria, www.rawfoodschef.com

Portabella Croquettes
Serves 6

Ingredients:

1½ cup almonds (soaked 10-12 hours)
1½ cup walnuts (soaked (10-12 hours)
1 cup pine nuts
3 portabella mushrooms diced and marinated in 2 Tbsp Nama Shoyu
       and ¼ cup olive oil
3 ribs of diced celery
¼ cup of red onion, minced
1/3 cup of cherry tomatoes, halved
1/3 cup of broccoli florets, small
1½ Tbsp thyme, dried
1½ Tbsp sage, dried
1/3 cup basil, fresh torn
3 Tbsp oregano, fresh, minced
2 Tbsp freshly-squeezed lemon juice
1 Tbsp chili powder
½ Tbsp Celtic sea salt
1 dash of cracked black pepper

To make:

Homogenize the nuts and seeds in a food processor with the S blade.

With the exception of the marinated portabella mushrooms, hand-mix the remaining ingredients with the homogenized nuts and seeds. The marinated, diced portabella mushrooms will be soft; toss them into the mix, including the excess marinade. Thoroughly hand-mix all ingredients.

Form into ½ dollar size patties and dehydrate at 105 degrees for 4-6 hours.

      Recipe by Chad Sarno, www.rawchef.com

Red Chili Croquettes with Cilantro Aioli
Serves 6

Ingredients for croquettes:

1 cup almonds, soaked 10-12 hours
1 cup walnuts, soaked 10-12 hours
½ cup sunflower seeds, soaked 10-12 hours
½ cup chopped cilantro leaves
1/3 cup diced red bell pepper
1/3 cup diced Fresno chilies (approx. 5 chilies)
3/8 cup diced yellow onion
¼ cup green onions, rough minced
3 Tbsp chopped parsley
4 cloves garlic
1 cup sun-dried tomatoes, soaked 1-2 hours
3 Tbsp dark miso
1½ Tbsp freshly-squeezed lemon juice
2 Tbsp olive oil

2 Tbsp minced jalapeno
2½ Tbsp chili powder
1 Tbsp cumin
1 tsp garlic powder
½ tsp onion powder
½ tsp Celtic sea salt or to taste
¼ tsp chipotle chili powder

Ingredients for Cilantro Aioli:
1½ cups Thai coconut meat
½ cup raw cashews, soaked
2 Tbsp olive oil
1 Tbsp freshly squeezed lemon juice
½ Tbsp date paste
2 cloves garlic
1 tsp chopped shallots
1 tsp unprocessed sea salt
2 Tbsp minced cilantro
chives to garnish

To make croquettes: Soak sun-dried tomatoes until they are very soggy. Place the soaked and rinsed almonds, walnuts, sunflower seeds, cilantro, and parsley in a food processor. Using the S blade, blend leaving a slightly chunky consistency. Remove nut mixture and place into a mixing bowl. Hand mix red bell pepper, Fresno chilies, onion, and green onion into the nut mixture and set aside.

Place the remaining ingredients into the food processor and blend into a thick paste. Add the paste to the nut mixture and hand mix thoroughly. Using a tablespoon, scoop out the mixture and form it into patties. Place patties onto a non-stick drying sheet and dehydrate at 145 degrees for 1 hour and then an additional 4 hours at 105 degrees. (To use as taco meat, just spread it onto a non-stick drying sheet and dehydrate.)

To make aioli: Blend all ingredients except cilantro until smooth. Hand mix in cilantro and chill before use.

To assemble: Using a pastry bag or squeeze bottle, place a dollop of aioli on top of each croquette. Sprinkle with chives.

Recipe by Joshua McHugh, www.livingintentions.com

Pesto Lasagna
Serves 8 to 12

Ingredients for the marinade:
4 cups pure water
1 cup cold-pressed extra-virgin olive oil
1 cup fresh basil, torn
¼ cup Nama shoyu
1 lemon, freshly-squeezed juice of
2 cloves garlic, minced or pressed
1 Tbsp ginger, grated

Ingredients for the vegetable layers:
1 yellow bell pepper, sliced thin

1 red bell pepper, sliced thin
1 orange bell pepper, sliced thin
3-4 portabella mushrooms, sliced thin
4 zucchini, sliced thin
4 yellow squash, sliced thin

Ingredients for the pesto:
½ cup pine nuts
4-5 cloves garlic
½ cup fresh cilantro
½ cup fresh basil
3 Tbsp Nama Shoyu
2 Tbsp freshly-squeezed lemon juice
2 cups tomato, chopped

Ingredients for the cheese dip:
2 cups cashews soaked for 4 hours or longer
2 cups pure water
1½ - 2 cups fresh dill
Herbamere seasoning salt

To marinade:
In a large bowl, mix together all of the ingredients for the marinade.

To make vegetable layers:
1. Add all of the ingredients for the vegetable layers to the bowl of marinade. Add in enough water to cover (a few cups).
2. Marinate for a couple of hours or overnight.
3. Drain the vegetables.

To make the cashew cream cheese dip:
1. Place half of the water into a blender and slowly add the cashews.
Add water as needed, until all of the cashews are gone. Keep this mixture thick by adding a few cashews at a time, until the blender is no longer able to turn over the mixture.
2. Add dill and Herbamere to taste.

To make the pesto:
1. Place all ingredients, except for the tomato, in a food processor and blend well until blended, but still chunky.
2. Add tomatoes and pulse chop a few seconds until well blended but not soupy.

To assemble:
1. In a lasagna pan, layer the zucchini on the bottom of the pan just slightly overlapping each other.
2. On top of the zucchini, layer the yellow squash in the same manner.
3. Pour pesto on top of squash and spread evenly the length of the pan.
4. On top of the pesto place another layer of the squash, (just one layer, alternating the two types of squash).
5. On top of the squash layer, place a layer of the mushrooms.
6. Pour dill cream cheese dip over the previous layers and spread evenly throughout the length of the pan.
7. Add another layer of squash on top of the dill cream cheese dip
8. Place a layer of all of the peppers on top of the squash.

Note: This lasagna is best when you let it stand for a few hours to allow the flavors to mingle. I've been making this dish for years. It's delicious, with a lighter taste than the cheese and sauce lasagna. Smooth and flavorful, this dish is also lovely to look at!

Recipe by Alissa Cohen, www.alissacohen.com

Walnut Mushroom Loaf
Serves 8

Ingredients:

2½ cups walnuts, soaked overnight and rinsed
½ cup almonds, soaked overnight and rinsed
1 cup pumpkin seeds, soaked overnight and rinsed
2 cups portabella mushrooms, marinated in Nama shoyu for 15 minutes
1½ cloves of garlic
¾ cup celery, chopped
1 cup red bell pepper, chopped
1¾ cup carrot pulp (what is left after juicing carrots) or rolled oats
½ cup yellow onion, chopped
1 jalapeno pepper, seeds removed
¼ cup fresh rosemary leaves
1 Tbsp ginger, minced
¼ cup dried parsley
1 tsp cumin powder
½ Tbsp Celtic sea salt
½ cup cold-pressed extra-virgin olive oil

To make:

Chop the vegetables first and mix all the ingredients in a bowl, add the onions last (use the mushrooms but not the shoyu).

In a high quality food processor, such as a Cuisinart, add 3-4 cups at a time and process until well blended. Scoop out ½ cup at a time and form that into a personal-sized loaf. Place the 8 loaves on a teflex or parchment paper covered dehydrator sheet. Dehydrate at 95 degrees for 6 hours. Serve and enjoy!

Recipe by Cilantro Live, www.cilantrolive.com

Vegetable Nut Loaf
Serves 4-6

Ingredients:

1 cup raw cashews or walnuts (soak walnuts 4 hours and rinse)
1 cup carrots, grated
1 cup celery, chopped to ¼ inch square pieces
1/4 cup cabbage, shredded
1/4 cup onion, Spanish or Vidalia
1/2 tsp garlic, minced
1/4 tsp thyme leaves, dry
1/4 tsp basil leaves, dry
1/4 tsp unprocessed sea salt
1/8 tsp black pepper

1 tsp freshly-squeezed lemon juice

To make:

1) Place nuts into food processor and run on high until smooth.
2) Place into large bowl.
3) Add remaining ingredients and mix well, adding water if necessary to make it hold together.
4) Press into a loaf pan and refrigerate at least 3 hours before serving.
   Recipe by Brad Wolff, Vegan Food Scientist/product developer; email: veganfoods@yahoo.com

Christina's Living Cashew Curried Veggies
Serves 4-6

Ingredients for curry sauce:

2 medium tomatoes

2 cloves of garlic or 1 tsp asafoetida powder

1 Tbsp freshly squeezed lemon juice

1 Tbsp raw agave or raw honey or one packet of stevia powder

1 Tbsp freshly grated ginger or ½ tsp powder (do not add more stivia or a bitter
   taste will occur)

1 Tbsp freshly grated turmeric or 1 tsp turmeric powder

1 tsp unprocessed sea salt

1 can of preservative-free coconut milk (cream of coconut) **or** the meat
   and some liquid (milk) from young coconuts totaling 13 oz. after blending (blend
   until the texture is that of heavy cream)

5 tsp curry powder

1 cup raw cashews that have been soaked from 4 to 6 hrs and rinsed

To make:

Place all ingredients, except cashews, in a food processor or blender and process until smooth.

Suggested use:

Pour curry mix over the following raw veggies or veggies of your choice and the soaked cashews.

Ingredients for Veggies:

½ bunch of broccoli, chopped into small pieces

½ head of cauliflower, chopped into small pieces

1 large tomato, diced

1 large red pepper, diced

¼ cup onion sprouts or any desired sprouts

½ sweet onion, finely chopped

2 Tbsp chopped leaks or scallions

¼ bunch of chopped cilantro

   Recipe by Christina Ott, www.barefootbuilder.com

Thai Vegetables in Coconut Sauce, "Phak Tom Kati"

Ingredients:

1 cup coconut cream (see Thai Coconut Yogurt recipe for directions on making)
½ cup garden peas
½ cup long beans (green beans), broken into 2" pieces
½ cup mushrooms, sliced
1 cup cabbage, shredded
2 Tbsp shallots or purple onions, sliced finely
1 Tbsp Nama Shoyu
1 Tbsp raw agave
1 Tbsp Habanero or Birdseye chilies, finely sliced
1 Tbsp green peppercorns
½ tsp lime zest (or shredded Kaffir lime leaves)

To make:

In a blender pour the coconut cream and mix in the agave, Nama shoyu, and lime zest. Add the shallots and pepper, and gently blend for 1-2 minutes until aromatic. Taste for the balance of sweet and salty, and adjust if necessary. Pour into a large bowl and add the vegetables. Allow to marinate for a few hours or overnight. Serve with either raw vegetable noodles or as is.

Recipe by Dorit, www.serenityspaces.org

Shrimp Brazil
Serves 4

Ingredients:

2 cups Brazil nuts, soaked in filtered water overnight
6 oz. young coconut meat
½ medium onion
½ tsp Celtic sea salt
¼ cup finely chopped cilantro
1 tsp minced garlic
1 tsp minced ginger

To make:

1) Drain and rinse the Brazil nuts.
2) In a food processor, blend first 4 ingredients until creamy.
3) Transfer to a bowl and add in by hand cilantro, garlic and ginger.
4) On an unbleached parchment paper or teflex-lined dehydrator tray, shape into shrimp-like figures and dehydrate at 95 degrees F for 4 hours, then turn over, remove teflex or parchment paper and continue to dehydrate for another 2 to 4 hours.

Recipe by Rhio, www.rawfoodInfo.com

Perfectly Healthy Pizza

Ingredients for crust:
Italian Essene bread for crunchy crust (see recipe earlier in this chapter)
or
Pizza Parlor Crust for soft crust (see recipe earlier in this chapter)

Ingredients for cheese: (makes enough for 4 slices)
1 cup raw almonds
½ tsp unprocessed sea salt
2 Tbsp freshly squeezed lemon juice

To make cheese:
Soak raw almonds for 12 to 24 hrs.
Rinse almonds and place them with lemon juice in a blender. Slowly add pure water until the water level is just under the level of the uppermost portion of the almonds, add the salt and process until creamy.
Spoon the mix onto the Essene bread and dehydrate at 100 degrees for about an hour.

Sauce:
After the cheese has dehydrated, spoon on the marinara sauce (see Veggie Noodle Marinara recipe in this chapter). Then let the sauce warm on top of the pizza in the dehydrator for ½ hr or so.

Toppings:
Add diced onions, tomatoes, olives, red peppers, sprouts and mushrooms (mushrooms are best when marinated in Nama shoyu for several hours) to taste.

Recipe by Craig Sommers, www.rawfoodsbible.com

Veggie Noodle Marinara
Serves 4-6

Ingredients for marinara sauce:
4 medium tomatoes
2½ Tbsp sun-dried tomato powder
¼ small red beet (the beet is to achieve a red colored sauce; without it, it does not look
     appealing)
¼ small red onion
2 cloves garlic or 1 tsp asafoetida powder
2 dates, pitted (optional)
2 Tbsp Italian seasoning (Frontier makes an organic one)
1¼ tsp unprocessed sea salt
1/8 tsp cayenne pepper
1 lemon, juice of
1 cup fresh basil (¼ cup chopped)
½ cup parsley (¼ cup chopped)

To make sauce:
Place ingredients in a food processor or blender and process.
Add chopped herbs near the end of blending for a chunky sauce.

Ingredients for noodles:
4 zucchinis, medium sized

Optional veggies for making noodles include beet, daikon radish, sweet potato, and jicama

To make noodles:

With a Spiral Slicer or a Spirooli, spin the zucchini into noodles. The spiral slicer makes angel hair style noodles and the Spirooli makes thicker noodles. Both of these machines make noodles that are very long. Enjoy the long noodles or cut them in half.

Add a splash of your preferred oil, sea salt, and a squeeze of citrus of choice to the noodles. Massage the noodles with your hands & fingers, After marinating for at least ten minutes, pour off the liquid and save it for use in another sauce, beverage, or soup base. Pasta is great the next day.

Optional topping: 2 Tbsp ground pine nuts

To serve:

Spoon the marinara on top of the veggie noodles and eat! For a change, try using Christina's curry sauce or her French dressing recipe on the vegetable noodles!

Recipe by Katherine Narava Kaufman, www.SimplyLovingRaw.com

Pasta with Alfredo Sauce
Serves 6

Ingredients for sauce:

1½ cups raw cashews, soaked for a few hours to soften

½ cup pine nuts

1 cup peeled and cubed zucchini (about ½ of a zucchini)

1½ Tbsp fresh oregano leaves, finely chopped, or 1¼ tsp oregano powder

¼ - ½ cup cold-pressed extra-virgin olive oil

½ - ¾ tsp Celtic sea salt

2 cloves garlic

1 tsp freshly-squeezed lemon juice

¼ cup fresh or soaked Shitake mushrooms (soak for 3-8 hours)

½ cup water from the soaking of dry shitake mushrooms if available (optional)

1½ cups pure water

2 scallions, finely chopped

3 baby Portabella mushrooms or ½ large Portabella mushroom sliced very thin

To make sauce:

Place all the sauce ingredients, except the scallions and baby Portabella mushrooms, into a high-powered blender and blend until very smooth and creamy.

Hand-mix the scallions and Portabella mushrooms into the sauce, sprinkling a few of the scallions on top for a garnish.

To serve:

Serve on vegetable pasta as described in the *Veggie Noodle Marinara* recipe. Zucchini noodles are especially good with this sauce. Peel the zucchini before you spiralize it.

Recipe by Christina Ott, www.barefootbuilder.com

Macaroni and Cheese
Serves 4-6

Ingredients:
2 large peeled yams
1½ cups pine nuts
2 Tbsp turmeric powder
¼ cup cold-pressed extra-virgin olive oil
1/3 cup pure water
½ tsp unprocessed sea salt (optional)
1 lemon, juice of
2 Tbsp unpasteurized mellow white miso (Hawaiian) for less salty flavor,
     or 3-4 Tbsp of any other unpasteurized miso for stronger flavor

To make macaroni:
Using a mandolin slicer, carefully make as many lengthwise thin slices as you can from the peeled yam. Then stack the slices and slice them into small rectangular shapes. Do this with both yams. Put the squares into a bowl or Pyrex glass pan. Drizzle with olive oil and squeeze the lemon juice on top. Sprinkle the sea salt on top and mix the yams until they are all covered in the olive oil mix. Set aside and allow to marinate.

To make nacho cheese sauce:
Blend all remaining ingredients in a Blend-Tec Champ HP-3 blender or any high speed blender. Then pour the sauce over the yams and mix evenly with a fork; the yams will get curly naturally.
Enjoy the dish right away or let it sit longer for a softer and more "cooked" taste. Refrigerate leftovers; they will last for a few days in the fridge.
     Recipe by Bryan Au, author of *Raw in Ten Minutes*

Bodacious Veggie Burgers
Makes about 12 burgers

Ingredients:
3½ cups carrot pulp from a juicer (not the juice)
3 cups Portabella mushrooms (chopped)
1 cup almonds (soaked overnight and rinsed)
½ cup sweet onion (chopped)
5 tsp minced garlic or 2 tsp asafoetida powder
¼ cup cold-pressed extra-virgin olive oil
4 Tbsp unpasteurized mellow white miso

To make:
Place the soaked almonds in a food processor using the S blade and process well. Mix all ingredients in a large bowl (including the processed almonds). Place half (or less) of the mixture in the food processor at a time and process until smooth. Mix the processed ingredients by hand in the bowl one more time to ensure an even mix. Form patties and place on parchment paper in the dehydrator at 100 degrees for as many hours as it takes to get to the desired hardness. Flip burgers after 6 hours.
     Recipe by Craig Sommers, www.rawfoodsbible.com

Buckwheat Gnocchi

Ingredients:

2 cups buckwheat, soaked
1 cup Brazil nuts or pecans, unsoaked
2 cups parsley or cilantro or spinach
1 Tbsp unprocessed sea salt (or to taste)
½ lemon, freshly pressed juice of
1-2 cups pure water

To make:

Place nuts in a blender with lemon juice, salt, and just enough water to cover the nuts. Blend to a creamy consistency. Add buckwheat and blend until smooth. The mixture needs to be thick, so add more nuts if the mixture is runny. Pour the mixture into a bowl. Cut the greens into very small pieces. This may be done in a food processor using the pulse button. Add the greens to the buckwheat dough and mix with a spoon.

Optional:

At this point you may add garlic, onions, or other spices, but authentic Italian gnocchis are kept very simple.

To complete:

Fill a large nozzled pastry bag with the mix and squeeze long strips onto a dehydrator screen. Cut the strips with a knife or spatula into desired sizes. With a spoon, press each gnocchi's in its center to give them a rounded shape.

Dehydrate for approximately 4 hours and serve warm with Creamy Garlic Sauce (see sauce section) or the sauce of your choice.

Recipe by Ursula Horaitis, www.goodmoodfood.com

Herbed Coconut Unturkey with Herb Stuffing
Serves 4

Ingredients:

1 cup red pepper, diced small
1 cup Brazil nuts (soaked 3 hours and rinsed)
½ cup fresh cilantro, chopped
¼ cup cold-pressed extra-virgin olive oil
1 tsp thyme powder
1 tsp sage powder
2 cloves garlic
1 tsp Celtic sea salt
1 cup corn off the cob
2 young Thai or green coconuts, cut the meat into medium-sized oval shapes

To make:

In a food processor with the S blade, process all the ingredients except the coconut meat and red pepper. Hand-mix the processed ingredients with the red pepper. Make a sandwich with the coconut pieces as the bread and the mixture as the filling. Warm in a dehydrator for 1-2 hours.

Recipe by Shanti Devi Michal; email: rawpeach25@yahoo.com

Bombshell Burritos
Serves 4

Ingredients for filling:

2 cups sunflower seeds, (unsoaked)
½ cup sun dried tomatoes, rehydrated
1 large tomato
1 tsp unprocessed sea salt
¼ teaspoon paprika powder
2 tsp cumin
6 Tbsp chili powder
¼ cup cold-pressed, extra-virgin olive oil
3 cups pure water

Ingredients for topping:

1 cup diced tomato
minced cilantro

Ingredients additional:

1 head romaine lettuce
Live "sour cream" (see Nondairy Cheeses section)
Guacamole

To make:

Grind sunflower seeds in blender. Blend remaining filling ingredients separately, add to ground seeds. Add more seeds if too runny or a little water if too thick. Best if it sits for a few hours in the fridge, covered. Spread mixture onto romaine leaves.
Top with guacamole, live "sour cream," diced tomatoes, and cilantro.

Recipe by Amy Rachelle, www.amyrochelle.com

Buttered Zucchini
Serves 2-4
Preparation time: 10 minutes

Ingredients:

4 cups zucchini or other squash, shredded
¼ cup pumpkin seeds, soaked in pure water for 6-12 hours
¼ cup sunflower seeds, soaked in pure water for 6-12 hours
¼ cup onion, chopped
1/8 cup cold-pressed extra-virgin olive oil (more or less if desired)
1 Tbsp dried basil
¼ tsp turmeric powder
½ tsp Himalayan crystal salt or other unprocessed sea salt
½ tsp black pepper

To make:

Place the shredded zucchini in a bowl. Add the remaining ingredients and toss.

Recipe by Nadhirrah; email nadhirrah@care2.com
Recipe taken from the book, *101½ Raw Zucchinis*.

Collard Chiffonade
Yields 2 cups

Ingredients:

12-15 small collard green leaves, or any dark leafy greens
2 Tbsp cold-pressed grapeseed oil
1 Tbsp cold-pressed walnut oil
1 pinch Celtic sea salt
¼ cucumber, sliced on angle
¼ yellow squash, sliced on angle
¼ zucchini squash, sliced on angle
2 Tbsp bok choi kim chi
4 leaves purslane or parsley sprigs
1 large navel orange, thinly sliced
1 large Meyer's lemon, thinly sliced
3 Tbsp shelled hemp seeds

To make:

1. Rinse well and de-stem all leaves (collard or greens of your choice)
2. Tightly roll and cut chiffonade style (tiny cuts) across the rolled leaves.
3. Place in glass or wooden bowl. Add oils and pinch of unprocessed sea salt. With both hands, massage leaves until they appear to be sautéed.

To serve:

On a 6-8 inch plate place (in 12 o'clock position) one orange slice and one lemon slice. Mound greens on top of citrus.
At 8 o'clock place angle cut cucumber, layer on top with yellow squash then zucchini.
At 6 o'clock arrange by choice the kim chi and purslane.
Sprinkle hemp seeds on top and garnish with an edible flower of your choice.
This dish is better when served shortly after preparation.

Recipe by Aqeel Kameelah of Nova Community School

South American LifeFood "Ceviche" Boats in Mango Chutney Glaze
Serves 4

Ingredients for ceviche:

10–12 fresh shiitake mushrooms
3-4 lemons or 4-5 limes, freshly-squeezed juice of
1½ tsp Celtic sea salt
1/2 tsp crushed black pepper
1½ Tbsp raw apple cider vinegar
1/2 red onion, finely chopped
1 handful fresh parsley or cilantro, finely chopped
1/8 cup of pure water
1 small clove garlic, finely chopped, (optional)

Ingredients for mango chutney:

½ ripe mango
1 tsp. raw unfiltered wildflower honey
1 green onion, finely chopped
¼ ripe avocado
1½ tsp. Celtic sea salt

Ingredient for boat:

4 leaves of romaine lettuce

To make ceviche:

Gently break off the stems of each shiitake mushroom. Discard the stems and slice each mushroom into thin strips. The mushrooms should resemble, in consistency and size, tiny squid or clam bites. Place in a medium sized bowl.

Place the finely chopped red onion on top of the mushrooms.

Add the fresh lemon or lime juice to the mushroom and onion mix.

Add the Celtic sea salt, black pepper, apple cider vinegar, and water.

Take the handful of chopped parsley or cilantro and add to the mix. Mix with a spoon and allow the ingredients to marinade for about ten to fifteen minutes while you make the chutney.

To make mango chutney:

Peel half of a ripe mango. Chop or cube and process in a small food processor using the S blade. Add the salt, honey, ¼ avocado, and finely chopped green onion. Process very lightly into a thick chutney consistency.

To assemble ceviche boats:

Cut leaves of romaine in half and place a helping of the ceviche on each leaf boat.

Top with the mango chutney and ENJOY!!!

Recipe by John Schott, of Sacred Symbiosis, www.sacredsymbiosis.com

Raw Vegan Bindi Masala with Spiced Basmati "Rice"

Ingredients for Bindi Masala:
3 cups okra, cut into very thin strips
3 cups sun dried tomatoes, soaked in pure water until they are soft and then cut in very small thin squares.
1 medium-sized onion, finely chopped. You can soak it in pure water for a while and then rinse to diminish the intensity of the onion flavor if desired
1 tsp ginger, diced and smashed with a mortar
1 tsp garlic, diced and smashed with a mortar
1½ tsp chili powder
1 tsp of each spice: garam masala, turmeric, cumin powder, coriander powder, unprocessed sea salt to taste

To make:
Hand mix all the ingredients in a bowl.

To serve:
The cooked version is usually eaten with chapatti (a thin whole wheat bread) or over Basmati rice. I suggest Essene bread or my raw vegan version of spiced bastmati "rice". It is very tasty, filling, and tastes pretty close to the cooked version.

Ingredients for Spiced Basmati "Rice":
1 cup peeled & chopped parsnip
1/3 cup raw pine nuts
2 tbsp unpasteurized vinegar (raw apple cider vinegar)
1 tbsp of raw agave nectar or raw honey
¼ tsp unprocessed sea salt
1 tsp black pepper
1 inch of cinnamon stick, chopped as fine as you can, mashed it in a mortar, or processed in a coffee bean grinder
5-6 cloves, mash them in a mortar or process in a coffee bean grinder

To make:
Process the parsnip and the pine nuts in a food processor with the S blade until it looks like rice. Make sure not to over process. In a mixing bowl, hand-mix all of the ingredients.

To serve: Hand mix the Spiced Basmati rice with your Bindi Masala and enjoy!
Recipe by Mariela Rodríguez-Munn.

Side Dishes

Cranberry Relish
Serves 10

Ingredients:
1½ pints cranberries (frozen are OK)
2 medium apples (preferably red skinned)
1 medium pear (preferably red)
20 pitted dates (preferably medjool)
1 medium tangerine or orange, peeled and sectioned
½ tsp stevia extract (90% steviasides) or ¼ cup raw agave
½ cup almonds, walnuts, or shredded coconut (nuts should be soaked several hours first, shredded coconut should be sugar free)

To make:
Put all ingredients in a food processor and run until finely chopped. If everything will not fit into your food processor, put the first 3 ingredients in first and run processor until finely chopped. Then add remaining ingredients and run until finely chopped.
For best flavor, refrigerate at least one hour before serving.
Brad's favorite variation is with pineapple and coconut.
Recipe by Brad Wolff, Vegan Food Scientist/product developer;
email: veganfoods@yahoo.com

Pico De Gallo (Spicy Mexican Salsa)
Serves 4

Ingredients:
8 Roma tomatoes or 4 large vine-ripe tomatoes, diced
½ medium red or sweet onion, diced
1 clove garlic, finely chopped
1 bunch cilantro, chopped
1or 2 fresh jalapenos, chopped
1 lime, juice of
½ tsp unprocessed sea salt

To make:
Toss all ingredients and wait for 1-2 hours before serving.
Recipe by Chuck Ott.

Kim Chi
Makes 1 quart

Ingredients:
1 pound/500 grams Chinese cabbage (napa or bok choi)
1 daikon radish or a few red radishes
1-2 carrots
1-2 onions and/or leeks and/or a few scallions and/or shallots (or more!)
3-4 cloves of garlic (or more!)

3-4 hot red chilies, or any form of hot pepper, fresh, dried or in a sauce (without chemical preservatives as they inhibit microorganisms that are needed for fermentation) or more, depending on how hot-peppery you like your food.

3 Tbsp/45 milliliters fresh-grated gingerroot (or more!)

4 Tbsp unprocessed sea salt

To make brine:

Mix a brine of about 4 cups (1 liter) of pure water and 4 Tbsp (60 milliliters) of sea salt. Stir well to thoroughly dissolve the salt.

Add Vegetables:

Coarsely chop the cabbage, slice the radish and carrots and then let them soak in the brine, covered by a plate or other weight to keep the vegetables submerged until soft, a few hours or overnight. You may add other vegetables if you like, such as snow peas.

Prepare spices:

Grate the ginger, chop the garlic and onion, remove the seeds from the chilies and chop or crush, or throw them in whole. Mix the spices into a paste. If medicinal foods such as seaweeds or Jerusalem artichokes are desired, now is the time to add them.

Drain brine:

Set aside the brine after draining it off of the vegetables. Taste vegetables for saltiness. Rinse if too salty and add more salt if you cannot taste salt (a couple of tsp., to taste).

Mix:

Mix the vegetables with the spice paste and stuff them into a clean quart-size jar, pressing down until brine rises. If necessary, add some of the brine that was set aside to submerge the vegetables. Weight the vegetables down with a smaller jar filled with water.

Let sit.

Let the kim chi ferment in a warm place for about one week. Taste the mix often as it ferments. Mold may appear on top of the mix where it is exposed to the air. This is normal; simply remove the mold as it will not damage the final product. After the kim chi is ripe, store in the refrigerator.

Recipe by Sandor Ellix Katz from his book, *Wild Fermentation: The Flavor, Nutrition, and Craft of Live-Culture Foods.*

Savory Seed Sauerkraut (Salt Free)
Makes 1 quart

Ingredients:

1 medium-sized head of cabbage (about 1¼ lbs)

1 Tbsp caraway seeds

1 Tbsp celery seeds

1 Tbsp dill seeds (not dill weed)

To make:

Chop the cabbage into thin strips. Grind all the seeds with a mortar and pestle. Mix the seeds with the cabbage by sprinkling the seed mix evenly over the shredded cabbage. Tamp the mix tightly into a glass jar (a quart-sized wide-mouth mason jar works well). Add a little water (about 1 cup) to bring the brine above the cabbage level. Use a smaller jar filled with water, which fits into the cabbage jar, as a weight to hold the cabbage under the water.

Taste the mix often as it ferments. Mold may appear on top of the mix where it is exposed to the air. This is normal; simply remove the mold as it will not damage the final product. After the Sauerkraut is ripe, store in the refrigerator.

Salt preserves the crunchiness of the cabbage and helps develop sour flavors during fermentation by restricting what kind of organisms can survive in it. It is recommended that you add 1-2 tsp of unprocessed sea salt for better taste, but salt is optional.

Recipe by Sandor Katz (inspired by Paul Bragg) from his book, *Wild Fermentation: The Flavor, Nutrition, and Craft of Live-Culture Foods.*

Naturally Fermented Dill Pickles
Yields 1 quart jarful

Ingredients:
1 quart-sized Mason jar full of pickling cucumbers
5 garlic cloves, crushed and cut
¼ tsp whole dill seeds
¼ tsp whole black peppercorns
¼ tsp coriander seeds
¼ tsp whole yellow mustard seed
1 Tbsp sun-dried hand-harvested sea salt
pure water

To make:
Fill a sterilized quart mason jar with pickling cucumbers (not too tight).
Add all remaining ingredients to the mason jar that is already filled with cucumbers.
Top off with the water.

Let the jar sit open (with no lid) at room temperature for about 10 days until the cucumbers are cured. The pickles are now ready. Close jar (with lid) and refrigerate to slow additional fermentation.

Recipe by Mark Wisdom, www.rawwisdom.com

Crêpes

Ingredients:
2 cups Brazil nuts or pecans, not soaked
1 cup golden flax seeds, ground and soaked for a few hours
5 pitted dates or ¼ cup raisins
1 lemon, freshly squeezed juice of
1 tsp cinnamon powder
1 tsp vanilla extract
1–2 cups pure water

To make:
Place dates or raisins in a blender with lemon juice, cinnamon, and vanilla. Then add the nuts and just a bit of water to assist in blending. Mix until a smooth consistency is reached, add the flax seeds and mix to achieve a dough-like consistency. If the dough is too liquid add some ground unsoaked flax seeds. If the dough is too thick, add more water.

Take an ice-cream scoop sized ball of dough and flatten it to a 6-7 inch pancake on your Teflex sheet or unbleached parchment paper. Dehydrate for about 2-3 hours. Then carefully take the crêpes off of the sheet or paper and place directly on the dehydrator screen. Dehydrate for another 1-2 hours. Remove the crêpes before they become crispy. They should keep their flexibility.

To serve: The crêpes may now be filled with fruit and cream as desired. (See Ricotta Cheese/Cream recipe for cream)

Variation: The crêpe recipe above is a sweet dish. If you desire a savory flavor, replace the dates (or raisins), cinnamon, and vanilla with the same amount of avocado and add unprocessed sea salt or Nama Shoyu to taste. The crêpes can now be filled with the vegetables of your choice.

Recipe by Ursula Horaitis, www.goodmoodfood.com

Fruit Haroset

Ingredients:
2 cups shredded coconut (unsweetened)
2 cups sunflower seeds, soaked for several hours first
1 cup raisins, soaked for at least an hour first
2 cups apples, diced or shredded
1 Asian pear, diced
½ cup dried figs, soaked to rehydrate and chopped first
¼ cup dried fruit soak water (left after soaking the figs and raisins)
2 tsp cinnamon
zest of 1 lemon
zest of 1 orange
2 tsp Himalayan salt (or Celtic sea salt)

To make:
Hand mix all the ingredients well and serve.
May be served with Almond milk.

Recipe by Tree of Life Café.

Un-Sautéed Greens
Serves 4

Ingredients:
2 bunches or 4 cups chopped kale, washed well in pure water
1/8-1/4 cup cold-pressed, extra-virgin olive oil
1 lemon, freshly squeezed juice of (equals 3 Tbsp)
1/2 tsp unprocessed sea salt

To make:
Stack the kale leaves so that each one nests into the one below it then roll them tightly together. Holding the roll firmly, cut it into thin slices as you would a sushi roll. Place the cut greens in a bowl. Coat the greens with the remaining ingredients. Massage well with both hands (infuse with love as the palms of the hands represent the Heart)
Optional: use any wild greens from nature's garden. Add soaked nuts or hemp seeds. Enjoy!

Recipe by Katherine Nirava Kaufman, www.simplylovingraw.com

Garlic MacMash Unpotatoes with Marvelous Mushroom Gravy
Serves 4-6

Ingredients for Mushroom Gravy:
1 cup fresh young coconut meat
½ avocado
2 cloves garlic
¼ cup red onion
1 tsp Celtic sea salt
¾ cup soaked dried or fresh Crimini mushrooms
1 tsp black pepper

Ingredients for Unpotatoes:
1 head cauliflower
3 cups macadamia nuts (soaked for 3 hrs)
2 lemons, juice of
3 cloves of garlic
½ tsp black pepper
1 tsp unprocessed sea salt

To make mushroom gravy:
In a food processor using the S blade, or in a blender, process all the ingredients until smooth, adding water until desired consistency is reached (1 cup works well).

To make unpotatoes:
Run the head of cauliflower and the soaked macadamia nuts through a food processor.
Add the garlic, sea salt, coarsely ground black peppercorns and lemon juice and mix well.

To serve:
Scoop out a clump of Unpotatoes and pour mushroom gravy on top.

Recipe by Shanti Devi Michal; email: rawpeach25@yahoo.com

Candied Yams
Serves 4

Ingredients:

4 yams or sweet potatoes, peeled

1 or 2 Tbsp raw honey or raw agave nectar

To make:

In a food processor, using the S blade, process the yams until smooth. Add sweetener a little at a time, processing each time you add, and then tasting until desired sweetness is reached. Be careful not to over-sweeten.

Recipe by Shanti Devi Michal, email: rawpeach25@yahoo.com

Wild Rice Pilaf
Serves 2

Ingredients:

1¼ cups wild rice that has been soaked at least 24 hours or until 1/3 of it has split

½ cup chopped red bell pepper (about 1 average-sized pepper)

2-3 Tbsp cold-pressed extra-virgin olive oil

2 Tbsp freshly-squeezed lemon juice

1 tsp Nama shoyu or 1 pinch Celtic sea salt

2-3 Tbsp chopped scallions

Optional Ingredients:

¼ - ½ cup raw cashews, chopped

1 Tbsp grated sweet onion

1 Tbsp nutritional yeast (for thick creamy sauce)

To make:

Hand mix all ingredients and serve.

Note: This dish is not for people with bad teeth because it is very chewy.

Recipe by Christina Ott and Craig Sommers, www.rawfoodsbible.com

Soups

Fresh Corner Gazpacho
Serves 8

Ingredients:
5 tomatoes, diced
1 small red pepper, cored, seeded and diced
1 small yellow pepper, cored, seeded and diced
¼ large zucchini, diced
½ large cucumber, quartered lengthwise and thinly sliced
¼ onion, diced
1 Tbsp chopped garlic
½ cup cold-pressed extra-virgin olive oil
¼ tsp cayenne pepper, or less to taste
¼ bunch parsley, washed, dried and coarsely chopped
3 Tbsp balsamic vinegar
2 Tbsp Spike (a blend of vegetables and salt sold in health food stores)

To make:
1. In a bowl, combine the tomatoes, red and yellow peppers, zucchini, cucumber, onion and garlic. Stir well. In a small bowl, combine the olive oil, cayenne, parsley, balsamic vinegar and Spike. Whisk together and pour over the veggies.
2. Ladle 1½ cups of the mixture into the jar of a blender. Blend on high until the mixture has liquefied. Pour back into the bowl and stir together.
3. Refrigerate until ready to serve.
Recipe by Karyn Calabrese, www.karynraw.com

Crème of Mushroom Soup
Serves 6-8

Ingredients:
½ cup raw cashews or raw macadamia nuts, soaked for a few hours in pure water
2 cups raw almonds, soaked overnight
4 cups button mushrooms
2/3 cup Nama Shoyu
4 medium-sized cloves of garlic
10 cups of pure water

To make:
First, blend nuts and water well until liquid is smooth and silky.
Then add in the rest of the ingredients and blend. (If you want your soup warm, use half the water in making the soup and then when serving, heat the other half of the water and add to the soup while stirring constantly.)

Recipe by Rod Rotondi, founder of Leaf Cuisine, www.leafcuisine.com

Carrot Ginger Soup
Serves 3

Ingredients:

1½ cups carrots, finely chopped

1 Tbsp unpasteurized white miso

1 tsp fresh ginger root, finely chopped

1 clove garlic

2 cups pure water

To make:

Blend all of the ingredients, except ¾ cup of the carrots. Pour the blended ingredients over the carrots and serve.

Great for building lung strength.

Recipe by Brigitte Mars, www.brigittemars.com

Creamy Cucumber Herb Bisque
Serves 4-6

Ingredients:

1 small leek

1 cucumber, chopped

1 zucchini, chopped

2-4 scallions, chopped

1 handful of fresh herbs of choice (dill or basil or cilantro, etc.)

1-2 Tbsp freshly squeezed lemon juice

1 Tbsp onion powder

1 tsp Celtic sea salt (or to taste)

½ - 1 avocado depending on desired thickness or ¼ - ½ cup raw cashews

4 cups pure water

To make:

Blend all ingredients except herbs until creamy. Top with minced herbs.

Recipe by Matt Samuelson; email: mattsamuelson@yahoo.com

Aiyah's Garden Living Corn Chowder
Serves 3-4

Ingredients:

2½ cups pure water

3 cups corn, fresh off the cob

1 cup avocado, mashed

¼ cup celery, diced

¼ cup onion, diced

1 Tbsp Nama Shoyu, or to taste

1 tsp ginger, peeled & minced

1 tsp garlic, minced (optional)

1 tsp unprocessed sea salt, or to taste

½ tsp jalapeño, seeded & minced

¼ tsp black pepper, ground to taste

1 pinch cayenne pepper

2 tsp cilantro, minced

½ cup red bell pepper, diced

To make:

1. Place 2 cups of corn and all remaining ingredients except cilantro and red bell pepper in a blender and blend until smooth.

2. Pour into serving bowls. Top with cilantro, bell pepper and remaining 1 cup of corn. Serve chilled. (30 min prep.)

Recipe reprinted from *Vegan World Fusion Cuisine* www.veganfusion.com, the cookbook and 'wisdom work' from the chefs of the Blossoming Lotus Restaurant on Kauai, HI. www.blossominglotus.com

Bouillabaisse (Hearty Sea Vegetable Stew)
Makes approximately 6, 8-oz. servings

Ingredients:

½ ounce each of the following dried seaweeds: silky sea palm, nori, armed, hijiki

1 tsp ground cumin

1 Tbsp freshly-squeezed lemon juice

1 cup raw tahini (blonde)

1 Tbsp raw black sesame tahini

1 tsp minced garlic

1½ tsp minced ginger

¼ cup ground golden flax seeds

1½ tsp minced sage

1½ tsp minced hyssop

½ - 1 tsp ground cayenne

1 Tbsp unprocessed sea salt

½ cup chopped yellow onion

1 Tbsp unprocessed coconut oil

4 ounces unpasteurized chickpea miso

1 quart pure water

To make:

With scissors, cut seaweed into small pieces.

Soak seaweed in 1 quart of water for 2 hours. (If preparing this dish for someone who dislikes the taste of fish, after soaking, pour off the soaking water into a measuring cup. Note how much liquid is there and discard, replace with fresh water. Rinse seaweed well)

Again, while suspended in water, cut the seaweed into small pieces as it will have swelled to greater size.

Place on gas burner, on lowest setting (I have used an electric burner with success).

Add the 8 ounces of chickpea miso. Stir until miso is dissolved. Add tahini and stir until dissolved. Stir in the rest of the ingredients.

Stir every so often. Warm to "finger hot" (mixture should be thick and creamy after fifteen minutes of gradual warming).

This is an "I can't believe it's raw and vegan" dish that could pass for a seafood stew in any gourmet restaurant!

Recipe by Bruce Horowitz; email: chef_sprout2001@yahoo.com

One Love Soup

Ingredients:

1 cup raw cashews, soaked for 1 hour
2 Tbsp cold-pressed extra-virgin olive oil
1 red bell pepper
1 bunch watercress or parsley
2½ cups coconut water
1 clove garlic
1 slice ginger
2 tsp unprocessed (sun-dried) sea salt
2 tsp cumin
2 tsp curry powder
2 tsp dill seed
1/2 cup sun-dried tomatoes

To make:

Blend all ingredients in a Vitamix or high speed blender for 2 minutes. Pour into bowls and garnish with fresh herbs of your choice, julienne or shredded vegetables, lemon juice, and a little more sea salt if desired. Then give thanks and love.

Recipe by Rawsheed, www.rawsheed.com

Marvelous Miso Soup

Ingredients:

3-4 Tbsp unpasteurized miso paste (buy organic or risk eating GMOs)
¾ cup nutritional yeast (not a raw product)
dulse powder, to taste (optional)
3 Tbsp unprocessed coconut oil
pure water
Several vegetables of your choice. Here are some suggestions:
2 shredded carrots
1 large tomato, chopped
2-5 green onions, sliced thin
½ onion, finely chopped
2 leaves of dinosaur kale, finely chopped
¾ cup of finely chopped parsley
1 red bell pepper, diced
2-4 leaves of Napa cabbage chopped
handful of arugula leaves

To make:

With a fork, mix the miso paste with a small amount of water, into a thin paste. Do the same with the nutritional yeast.

Add the vegetables to the miso paste and nutritional yeast. Add just enough water to cover the veggies. Mix well and let it stand for several hours so the salt in the miso will draw water out of the veggies to simulate cooking.

Mix the soup with the liquefied coconut oil and serve.

Recipe by Christina Ott, www.barefootbuilder.com

Cambells Cream of Mushroom Soup
Serves 4-6

Ingredients:

1½ cups raw cashews
½ cup pine nuts
1 cup peeled and cubed zucchini (about ½ of a zucchini)
1½ Tbsp fresh oregano leaves or 1 tsp oregano powder
¼ - ½ cup cold-pressed extra-virgin olive oil
½ - ¾ tsp Celtic sea salt
2 large cloves of garlic
1½ Tbsp freshly squeezed lemon juice
2½ cups pure water or enough to achieve desired thickness
2 scallions, finely chopped
9 baby Portabella mushrooms

To make:

Place all the ingredients, except the scallions and 3 of the baby Portabella mushrooms, into a high powered blender and blend until very smooth and creamy. Slice the 3 remaining mushrooms very thin and hand mix them, along with the chopped scallions, into the soup. Sprinkle some chopped scallions on top as a garnish. Enjoy!

Recipe by Christina Ott, www.barefootbuilder.com

Cream of Celery Soup
Serves 4-6

Ingredients:

5 cups celery, de-stringed and coarsely chopped
1½ cups celery, de-stringed and finely diced
3 scallions, coarsely chopped
3 dried shiitake mushrooms, soaked 3-8 hours
½ cup soak water from shiitake mushrooms
3 cloves garlic
¼ cup pine nuts
¾ cup raw cashews
1 cup pure water
½ cup onion
½ large Portabella cap or 3 baby Portabellas
1 tsp unprocessed sea salt or to taste
¼ cup cold-pressed extra-virgin olive oil
¼ tsp oregano powder

To make:

Place cashews, pine nuts, 5 cups coarsely chopped celery, and water in a high speed blender or food processor; using the S blade, process until smooth. Add the rest of the ingredients excluding the 1½ cups finely chopped celery, and again, process until smooth. In a mixing bowl, hand-mix the remaining celery into the soup. Serve right away or chill and serve later.

Recipe by Christina Ott, www.barefootbuilder.com

Thai Curry Soup
Serves 2

Ingredients:
3 cups Thai coconut water (approx 1½ - 2 coconuts)
3 cloves peeled garlic
2 inch piece peeled ginger
1/4 cup freshly-squeezed lemon juice
1/4 cup cold-pressed extra-virgin olive oil
1/4 cup Nama Shoyu
1 Tbsp curry powder

To make:
1. In a blender, combine all the ingredients and thoroughly blend.
2. Pour into a serving bowl.
3. Using a ladle, remove and discard any foam that rises to the top.

Optional Garnish:
Chopped avocado
Chopped chives
Chopped tomato
Chopped red bell pepper
Chopped basil leaves
Chopped mint leaves
Chopped cilantro

Recipe by Matt Amsden, www.rawvolution.com

Tantalizing Lavender and Lemongrass Soup
Yields approximately 12 cups

Ingredients:
5 Tbsp lime juice, freshly squeezed
2 Tbsp lavender flowers, (soaked in warm water for 15 minutes)
1 entire lemongrass stalk, peeled and blended
4 cups young coconut meat
4 cups young coconut water
4 cups pure water
2 Tbsp Nama Shoyu
2 Tbsp curry powder
½ tsp cayenne powder
2 ground Thai chilies
Ground black pepper, to taste
1 tsp green leaf stevia
Unprocessed sea salt, to taste

To make;
Place all ingredients in a blender and blend until warm to the touch.
Garnish with cilantro and enjoy.

Recipe by Shakti Parvati, www.shaktiandthebluelotus.com

Cool Cucumber Soup
Serves 4-6

Ingredients:

5 Tbsp lemon juice, freshly squeezed
5 Tbsp fresh onion, chopped
5 cups of pure water
1½ avocados (Hass)
½ cucumber – remove seeds and dice
5 tsp of chopped cilantro
Dulse flakes

To make:

Place the first four ingredients in a high speed blender and blend until creamy (if using a Vita-mix, mix, blend at low speed for about 10 seconds). Pour the Avocado broth in soup bowls and add the diced cucumber and chopped cilantro. Sprinkle with Dulse flakes
Are you in the mood for a cool, delicious soup that is refreshingly alive? Here's the ticket! As always, organic vegetables are the best to use!
Serve right away for the best taste!
  Recipe by Elizabeth Michael.

Savory Squash Soup
Serves 6

Ingredients:

½ spaghetti squash
2 large cloves garlic
½ medium-sized yellow onion
1 medium-sized tomato
4 stems parsley
1 Tbsp unpasteurized miso (red)
½ cup raw tahini (unsalted)
½ cup cold-pressed extra-virgin olive oil
1 lime, freshly squeezed juice of
1 Tbsp oregano flakes
2 cups pure water

To make:

Peel the spaghetti squash and cut into pieces that will fit into the throat of your food processor. With the shedder blade, shred the squash. Set aside 3 cups of the shredded squash and cover the rest with pure water and 2 Tbsp of unprocessed salt for about 10 minutes (stir the salt in well). After 10 minutes is up, drain the squash and rinse lightly.
With the S blade of the food processor, process the remaining 3 cups of shredded squash, garlic, onion, tomato, parsley, oregano, and miso.
With a fork, mix the olive oil, lime juice, and tahini together.
Combine all the ingredients in a mixing bowl.
Serve with chopped parsley sprinkled on top as a garnish.
  Recipe by Christina Ott, www.barefootbuilder.com

Horizontal K's Green Curry Soup
Serves 4-6 hungry folks

Ingredients:

2 cups raw almonds, soaked 12 hours or more

2 or 3 fresh young coconuts

1 bunch organic cilantro

½ bunch organic green kale

½ head organic green cabbage

4 ribs organic celery

1 organic cucumber

1 organic carrot

1 organic zucchini

1 lime, freshly-squeezed juice of

1 thumbnail-sized chunk organic ginger

1 Tbsp extra-virgin organic coconut oil

1 tsp raw organic agave nectar

¼ tsp organic cayenne pepper

¼ tsp Himalayan Crystal Salt

To make:

Step 1. Julienne (slice thinly) the carrot, zucchini, ¼ head of cabbage, ¼ bunch of green kale, and one rib of celery. Combine in a bowl and set aside.

Step 2. Take a small handful of almonds and a ¼ of the cilantro and mince them. Set aside.

Step 3. Open the coconuts and pour the water into a vessel. Open them the rest of the way and scrape out the meat or jelly. Set aside.

Step 4. Run through your juicer the ginger, the remaining cilantro, the rest of the kale, cabbage, celery and the cucumber.

Step 5. In your blender combine the remaining almonds, coconut oil, cayenne, salt, agave nectar, coconut meat, and enough coconut water to blend. Blend thoroughly.

Step 6. In a big pot combine the juice with the blended mixture and any remaining coconut water. Stir until reaching a nice consistency.

Step 7. Ladle soup into bowls, and then top each bowl with a handful of julienned vegetables and a sprinkle of minced cilantro and almonds.

Note: Sounds like a lot when you read it, but it should only take you 20 minutes if you are a clear-headed, focused individual. It's well worth the effort. Cleaning the juicer is probably the most time-consuming part. I choose for it to be a meditation. Of course, there are plenty of substitutions that would work with this recipe. Add or subtract the veggies of your choice. Adding a clove of garlic to the juice works well, too.

Recipe by Keith Wahrer, www.barakafoods.com and www.dailyjuice.org

Salads

Awesome Carrot Salad
Serves 4-6

Ingredients:
3 lbs carrots, grated
2 celery ribs, diced
1 red bell pepper, chopped
1 small sweet onion, diced
1 large tomato, diced
2 tsp kelp powder
1¼ cup almond mayo (see recipe in condiments section)
1 pinch unprocessed sea salt (or to taste)

To make:
Mix all ingredients together and serve.
Recipe by Gentle World, www.gentleworld.org

Citrus, Avocado, and Mango Salad
Serves 2-4

Ingredients salad:
½ lb Mesclun salad mix (mixed baby greens)
1 large avocado, diced
1 large mango, diced
1-2 oranges, segmented and chopped (remove seeds)
1 grapefruit (optional), segmented and chopped (remove seeds)
¾ of a pint of cherry tomatoes
½ medium onion, sliced or diced
1 handful of chopped walnuts (soaked overnight and rinsed)
1 handful of pine nuts

Ingredients dressing:
¼ cup cold-pressed extra-virgin olive oil
½ lemon, freshly squeezed juice of
½ tsp prepared Dijon mustard or Magical Mustard from Condiment section
1 dash of dried or fresh thyme
1 dash of Celtic sea salt

Ingredients garnish:
paprika powder

To make:
1. In a large bowl place the Mesclun salad mix, avocado, mango, oranges, grapefruit, tomatoes and onion. Toss to mix and set aside.
2. Mix all the dressing ingredients in a small bowl.
3. Pour the dressing over the salad and toss well.
4. Serve the salad on plates and top with walnuts and pine nuts.
Garnish: Sprinkle paprika powder around the border of the plate.
Recipe by Rhio, www.rawfoodinfo.com

Carica Passionata
Serves 6

Ingredients:

5½ cups (1 medium-sized) unripe (green) papaya (see fruit section for explanation of unripe papaya)

1/3 cup passionfruit juice from ripe passionfruit (approx. 5 fruits)

2-4 Tbsp dulse flakes or unprocessed sea salt to taste

1 onion, finely chopped

5 cloves garlic, minced

3/4 cup cilantro, finely chopped

To make:

Peel and grate the papaya. Blend the pulp and seeds of the passion fruits in a blender. Strain through a wire sieve and discard the seeds. Mix all the ingredients and let it marinate for 1-3 hours. Decorate the perimeter of the dish with edible leaves (for example, spring mix). Place a small edible flower in the center (dandelion, nasturtium…) Serve with Love and enjoy sharing!

Recipe by Kitzia Howearth, www.alwaysseeds.org

Broccoli Miso Salad

Ingredients:

3 cups chopped broccoli (including the peeled stems)

1 cup chopped carrots

2 cloves garlic

3 Tbsp raw, unsalted tahini

3 Tbsp chickpea miso

3 Tbsp freshly squeezed lemon juice

2 Tbsp pure water

To make:

First peel the broccoli stems and then chop the broccoli stems and florets into small pieces in the food processor using the S blade. Don't chop this so much that it is mushy. Leave it in small bite-sized pieces. Take out and put into a bowl.

Next chop the carrots in the food processor. Take out and put in the bowl with the broccoli. Don't chop the broccoli and carrots together at the same time as the broccoli will become mushy before the carrots are chopped finely enough.

Next put the garlic in the food processor and chop. Then add the raw tahini, chickpea miso, water, and lemon juice into the food processor and blend all together. You do not have to clean out the food processor of the broccoli and carrots before you make the dressing. Just put it all in and whatever residue of broccoli and carrots are left in the processor will be blended up in the dressing.

Take the dressing out of the food processor and mix with the broccoli and carrots and toss well until all is coated.

Serving suggestions:

Serve on a bed of mixed baby greens and enjoy!

Recipe by Brenda Cobb, www.livingfoodsinstitute.com

Party Tabooli Salad
Serves 15–20

Ingredients:
5–6 bunches of parsley (6 small or 5 large), chopped
8 green onions (scallions), diced
½ cup quinoa soaked in pure water for at least 2 hours and drained
5 large tomatoes
½ to 1 red onion (½ if large or 1 if small), diced
1 Tbsp dried mint or 1 bunch of fresh peppermint, minced
1 cup cold-pressed extra-virgin olive oil
1 cup freshly squeezed lemon juice
1 Tbsp Celtic sea salt

To make:
Place all solid ingredients in a mixing bowl. Pour liquid ingredients and salt over the salad and mix well.

To serve:
Place a scoop of the salad on top of a Romaine lettuce or cabbage leaf. Enjoy!
Recipe by Omar Pure Heart of Live Cuisine, www.OmarsRawFood.com

Gourmet Bean Salad
Serves 2-4

Ingredients:
2 cups sprouted beans (French and red lentils, green peas and chickpeas)
Ingredients for sauce:
3 Tbsp raw tahini
2 tsp apple cider vinegar
1 Tbsp unprocessed coconut oil
½ lemon, juice of
¾ tsp grated ginger
1 pinch Celtic sea salt (optional)
½ tsp raw honey or raw agave syrup or 1 packet stevia
2½ Tbsp pure water

To make:
Hand mix all the ingredients for the sauce (if coconut oil is solid, heat it until it liquefies). Mix the sauce with the thoroughly rinsed beans and serve.
Recipe by Christina Ott and Craig Sommers, www.rawfoodsbible.com

Creamed Spinach
Yields 4-6 servings

Ingredients:
1 pound spinach chopped in food processor with the S blade
1-2 oz. of dehydrated almond meal (to make almond meal, soak the almonds in pure water overnight. Dehydrate them until the almonds are dry. Process the almonds in a food processor with the S blade until they resemble meal.)
4 yellow crooked neck squash, shredded

Ingredients for the sauce:

1½ ounces lemon juice, freshly-squeezed
5 ounces pure water
1½ cup pine nuts, soaked and rinsed
1½ cloves garlic
½ Tbsp kelp powder
1 pinch cayenne
1 tsp oregano

To make:

Blend the ingredients for the sauce in a blender thoroughly until creamy.

To serve:

Place the spinach in bowl. Pour the sauce over the spinach as desired and top with shredded yellow squash.

Sprinkle dehydrated almond meal on the top.

> Recipe by Ken Fisher.

Aggie's Italian Olive Salad

Ingredients:

½ large sweet onion, grated or (3 green onions, finely chopped)
15 ounces of pitted black olives (I suggest buying all olives from bulk sources or from glass jars and not from cans.)
10 ounces of pitted green olives
2 red peppers, diced
½ jar capers, rinsed well, optional (not preserved with distilled vinegar.)
3 ribs celery, trimmed, strings removed, cut into 1 inch pieces
3 stems flat Italian parsley
½ Tbsp dried oregano
3 large cloves of garlic
2½ Tbsp raw apple cider vinegar
Extra-virgin cold-pressed olive oil

To make:

Place all the solid ingredients in a food processor. Pulse the mix with the S blade to achieve a chunky mix. **Do not over-process.** Place the mix into a large bowl and add 2½ Tbsp of apple cider vinegar. Stir well. Saturate with olive oil. Place the olive salad into a jar, then top off with more olive oil. Refrigerate any unused portion and use within one week.

> Recipe by Agnes Adkison.

Apple Fennel Salad with Lemon Zest
Serves 4

Ingredients:

2 cups fennel, julienned thinly
2 cups apples, julienned thinly
1 Tbsp lemon zest
2 Tbsp freshly squeezed lemon juice
2½ Tbsp cold-pressed, extra-virgin olive oil
1½ Tbsp thyme, fresh and minced
1 Tbsp red jalapeno, seeded and minced
1 Tbsp Celtic sea salt
1 dash cracked black pepper

To make:

In a medium-sized mixing bowl, toss all ingredients well. Serve chilled.
A great variation can be to omit the apples and add tangerine slices instead.

Recipe by Chad Sarno, www.rawchef.com

Mother Grain Salad
Serves 4-6 people

Ingredients:

1½ cups sprouted quinoa (during sprouting, rinse 2-3 times per day, wait until a short tail is visible before preparing dish, 3 - 5 days)
7 sprigs parsley, chopped
1 cup cilantro, finely chopped
15-18 small capers, whole
¼ cup olives, pitted, your choice
1 large red pepper, julienne, marinated in cold-pressed extra-virgin olive oil
Nama Shoyu to taste (add a tiny amount at a time)
2 small ribs celery, ½ inch cuts
4-5 small cloves garlic, chopped fine
4 Tbsp cold-pressed walnut oil
3 Tbsp lemon juice, freshly-squeezed

To make:

Thoroughly rinse the quinoa. In a glass or wooden bowl, toss all ingredients.

To serve:

Place a large butter lettuce leaf or a banana leaf on a flat plate and place a scoop of the salad on top.

To garnish:

Place sprigs of lavender or edible flowers of your choice on top of each serving.
Note: Quinoa is known as the mother or super grain. This dish may be hard to chew for people with bad molars.

Recipe by Aqeel Kameelah of Nova Community School.

Cesar Salad
Dressing will cover 2–3 heads of lettuce

Ingredients for dressing:

1 cup cold-pressed extra-virgin olive oil

1 cup pure water

1 heaping Tbsp unpasteurized white mellow miso

2 – 3 cloves garlic

1 pitted date (medjool suggested) unless the olive oil is bitter, then use 2 dates

Ingredients for salad:

Romaine lettuce

Ingredients for parma-pine cheese:

1 cup pine nuts

1 Tbsp flax oil

¼ tsp Celtic sea salt

To make dressing:

Place half of the water and all remaining ingredients for the dressing in a blender and blend until smooth. Add a small amount of water and blend if needed to achieve desired consistency.

To make parma-pine cheese:

In a food processor, using the S blade, pulse all parma-pine cheese ingredients until you have a crumbly texture.

To assemble salad:

Place shredded lettuce in a bowl and toss with dressing. Sprinkle parma-pine cheese on top and serve.

Recipe by Blessing, email: blessingsalive@SBCglobal.net

Dressings

Christina's Creamy French Dressing
Serves 2-4

Ingredients:
¼ cup pure water
1/3 cup raw apple cider vinegar
1/3 cup cold-pressed extra-virgin olive oil
¼ tsp unprocessed sea salt (optional)
2-3 Tbsp raw agave or raw honey
2½ Tbsp cold-pressed, unrefined sesame oil (for best taste), or flax oil (for higher nutrition).
2 large cloves garlic, finely minced
1 cup nutritional yeast (not a raw product)

To make:
Put all **liquid** ingredients and garlic in a jar and shake to mix. Then add half of the yeast and shake until creamy. Add the other half of the yeast and shake again until thoroughly mixed.

This dressing is good right away but it is much better if you let it sit overnight, allowing the garlic flavor to mellow and mix with the rest of the dressing.

Recipe by Christina Ott, www.barefootbuilder.com

Tomato Dill or Basil Dressing

Ingredients:
3-4 medium tomatoes, chopped
2 Tbsp red onion, chopped
½ - ¾ cup fresh dill or basil (packed tightly), chopped
¼ cup cold-pressed extra-virgin olive oil
1 tsp Celtic sea salt
1-2 pitted dates
1 dash cayenne

To make:
In a food processor using the S blade, blend until smooth. For more texture, reserve ½ of the herbs until the end and blend lightly.

Variation: Add ½ avocado and ¼ - ½ cup of pure water for thicker, creamier dressing.

Recipe by Matt Samuelson; email: mattsamuelson@Yahoo.com

Salt-Free Creamy Tahini Dressing
Yields 2½ cups

Ingredients:
1/2 cup raw tahini (for a salt-free dressing, use unsalted raw tahini)
1/2 cup freshly-squeezed lemon juice (for sweeter dressing, use orange and lemon juice)
1/4 tsp coriander powder
1/8 tsp chili powder (optional)

½ cup cold-pressed, extra-virgin olive oil
1 tsp raw apple cider vinegar (optional)
¾ cup pure water
2 cloves garlic
1 or 2 Tbsp raw agave or raw honey or 1 packet stevia (do not add more stevia or it will taste bitter)

To make:

Place all ingredients in a blender and process until smooth.
Use more water or oil for a thinner dressing.
    Recipe by Christina Ott, www.barefootbuilder.com

Tahini Dressing
Yields one pint

Ingredients:

½ cup raw sesame tahini
½ cup cold-pressed, extra-virgin olive oil
4 limes or 3 lemons, freshly squeezed juice of
1 tsp mustard powder
3 garlic cloves
1 tsp Celtic Sea salt
3/4 cup water or rejuvelac (see beverage section for recipe)

To make:

In a blender, process until desired consistency is reached. Add more water if necessary and always add more garlic and salt till you love it and want to eat it on everything. Sesame seeds are a great source of Calcium.
    Recipes by Deva Khalsa, www.thecleanse.com

Avocado Dressing
Yields 2 cups

Ingredients:

¼ cup cold-pressed, extra-virgin olive oil
¼ cup fresh basil
1 clove garlic, minced
½ Tbsp fresh herbs of choice
¼ tsp onion powder
1/8 tsp cayenne pepper (optional)
¼ cup avocado
2 Tbsp nutritional yeast
1 cup pure water
2 Tbsp freshly-squeezed lemon juice
unprocessed sea salt to taste

To make:

In a blender, blend all ingredients until creamy. Serve fresh.
    Recipe by Gentle World, www.gentleworld.com

Sauces

Creamy Garlic Sauce

Ingredients:

2 cups macadamia nuts or cashews or blanched almonds
2-3 cups pure water (start with 2 and add more water if thinner sauce is desired)
1 lemon, freshly pressed juice of
2-3 cloves garlic (or to taste)
1-2 Tbsp Nama Shoyu or a dash of sea salt (to taste)

To make:

Place all ingredients in a blender and blend until smooth. If the sauce is too thick add more water. If the sauce is too thin add psyllium husk powder.

Variations:

Instead of garlic add marjoram or lavender or sun-dried tomatoes or mushroom.
Recipe by Ursula Horaitis, www.goodmoodfood.com

Buena Fortuna Curry Sauce
Serves 6

Ingredients:

1½ cups coconut cream
1 cup chopped cilantro (approx 1 bunch)
5 average-sized cloves of garlic or more
1 onion, chopped
1 Tbsp turmeric powder
1 pinch to 1 tsp cayenne powder
½ tsp unprocessed sea salt
50 fresh or dried curry leaves
¼ cup cold-pressed extra-virgin olive oil
½ tsp coriander (optional)

To make:

To make coconut cream, place coconut milk and meat in a blender and blend
until smooth (approx 1 brown coconut).
In a blender, mix curry leaves and olive oil until smooth. Add remaining ingredients and blend until smooth.

Serving suggestions: Pour over sprouted grains, shredded green papaya, or any shredded vegetables such as jicama, celery root, zucchini, beet root, or carrots.
Recipe by Kitzia Howearth; email: kitzia@siempresemillas.org

Condiments

Almond Mayo
Yields 1¼ cups

Ingredients:

1 cup raw almonds that have been soaked overnight
¾ cup pure water
1 Tbsp onion powder
1 tsp unprocessed sea salt
2-3 dates, pitted
1 lemon, juice of
1 dash raw apple cider vinegar
1/8 cup extra-virgin, cold-pressed olive oil

To make:

In a food processor using the S blade (or with a strong blender), thoroughly blend the almonds and water. Add the remaining ingredients, except the oil, and process. Slowly add oil (or extra water) while processing until the mixture becomes thick and smooth. Keep refrigerated and use as soon as possible.

Recipe by Gentle World, www.gentleworld.org

Nature's Gourmet Catsup
Yields 1½ cups thick catsup

Ingredients:

½ cup chopped tomatoes
¼ cup powdered sun-dried tomatoes (a coffee grinder works well to powder the sun-dried tomatoes if your store does not carry them)
1 clove garlic or ¼ tsp asafoetida powder
¼ cup chopped sweet onion
1 Tbsp cold-pressed, extra-virgin olive oil
4 tsp raw agave or raw honey or 1 pack stevia powder (do not add more stevia or it will taste bitter)
¼ tsp unprocessed sea salt
½ tsp Nama Shoyu
2 Tbsp raw apple cider vinegar
½ tsp nutritional yeast (optional)
5 Tbsp water for thick catsup (more for thin)

To make:

In a food processor, using the S blade, blend all ingredients until smooth.
Keep refrigerated.

Recipe by Craig Sommers, www.rawfoodsbible.com

Magical Mustard
Yields 1½ cups (approx.)

Ingredients:

1 cup yellow mustard seeds soaked overnight (sprouting optional)

½ cup raw apple cider vinegar

½ tsp unprocessed sea salt

½ tsp turmeric powder or 1 Tbsp diced root

To make:

In a blender or food processor using the S blade, process all ingredients until smooth. If needed, add pure water until the desired consistency is reached.

Keep refrigerated.

Recipe by Craig Sommers, www.rawfoodsbible.com

Chapter 9: Resources

Recommended Reading

- *Conscious Eating* by Gabriel Cousens, M.D.
- *Spiritual Nutrition* by Gabriel Cousens, M.D. (2005 edition)
- *Rainbow Green Live Cuisine* by Gabriel Cousens, M.D.
- *Sun Food Diet Success System* by David Wolfe (motivation to go raw)
- *Eating for Beauty* by David Wolfe (great Kirlian images)
- *12 Steps To Raw Foods* by Victoria Boutenko (how to go raw)
- *Raw Family* by the Boutenko's (a story of awakening)
- *Enzyme Nutrition* by Dr. Edward Howell (the science behind enzyme therapy)
- *The Essene Gospel of Peace, Book 1* translated by Edmond Bourdeoux Szekely (2000-year-old teachings that science holds true today)
- *Hippocrates Health Program* by Brian Clement
- *Living Foods for Optimum Health* by Brian Clement
- *Staying Healthy in an Unhealthy World* by Brian Clement
- *Raw Food Treatment of Cancer* by Kristine Nolfi, M.D.
- *Reclaiming Our Health,* Exploding the Medical Myth and Embracing the Source of True Healing by John Robbins
- *The Food Revolution,* How Your Diet Can Help Save Your Life And Our World, by John Robbins (I recommend the audio version)
- *Don't Drink Your Milk* by Frank A. Oski, M.D.
- *How to Grow Fresh Air* by Dr. B. C. Wolverton
- *The Sprouting Book* by Ann Wigmore (how to sprout)
- *Common Sense Health and Healing* by Dr. Robert Schulz
- *Water the Ultimate Cure by* Steven Meyerowitz

Books on Children and Living Foods

- *Raw Kids* by Cheryl Staycoff (transitioning children to raw foods)
- *Introduce Living Foods to Your Child* by Beth Montgomery (Guidebook for babies through two years)
- *Primal Mothering in a Modern World* by Hygeia Halfmoon, Ph.D.
- *Hallelujah Kids* by Julie Wandling (Christian perspective)
- *Eating Without Heating* by Sergei and Valia Boutenko (recipes)
- *Disease Proof Your Child* by Joel Furhman, M.D. (Not a raw food book but contains important information)

Recipe Books

- *Living on Live Food* by Alissa Cohen
- *Uncooking With Jamey & Kim* by Jamey Dina, N.D. and Kim Sproul, N.D.
- *Hooked On Raw* by Rhio
- *The Raw Truth* by Rene Underkoffler and Jeremy Saffron
- *Raw The UNcook Book* by Juliano
- *The Raw Gourmet* by Nomi Shannon
- *Kitchen Garden Cookbook* by Steve Meyerowitz
- *Living in The Raw* by Rosa Lee Calabro
- *Raw* by Roxanne Klein and Charlie Trotter
- *Elaina's Pure Joy Kitchen* by Elaina Love
- *The Raw Food Primer* by Suzanne Alex Ferraia
- *Living Cuisine* by Renee Loux-Underkoffer
- *Vital Creations* by Chad Sarno
- *Raw Foods Bible* by Craig B. Sommers
- *Thank God for Raw* by Julie Rodwell
- *The Complete Book of Raw Food* by Lori Baird and Julie Rodwell
- *Raw Cookery* by Roxie Olson
- *The Raw Food Primer* by Alex Febbara
- *Sunfood Cuisine* by Frederic Patenaude
- *How We All Went Raw* by Charles Nungesser and Stephen Malachi
- *The Delights of Living Food* by Jalissa Letendre
- *Recipes for Longer Life* by Ann Wigmore
- *Rawsome* by Brigitte Mars
- *The Art of Raw* by Ani Phyo
- *In The Season Thereof* and *A Season for Everything* by Nadhirrah
- *The Living Foods Lifestyle* by Brenda Cobb
- *Warming up to Living Foods* by Elysa Markowitz
- *Recipes for Life from God's Garden* by Rhonda J. Malkmus
- *The Joy of Living Live* by Zakah
- *Everyday Wholesome Eating* by Kim Wilson
- *Gods Way to Ultimate Health* by Dr. George Malkmus with Michael Dye
- *Raw Food Real World* by Mathew Kenny and Sarma Melngailis

Websites

WWW.RawFoodLife.com

WWW.RawFoods.com

WWW.RawFoodPlanet.com

WWW.RawFood.com

WWW.RawFoodsBible.com

WWW.RawFoodInfo.com

WWW.RawChef.com

WWW.RawFoodChef.com

WWW.PureJoyLivingFoods.com

WWW.SunWarrior.com

WWW.RawFoodResearch.com

WWW.EatRaw.com

WWW.RawFood.com

WWW.WigmoreDiet.com

WWW.Live-Food.com

WWW.KarynRaw.com

WWW.OneLuckyDuck.com

WWW.Live-Live.com

WWW.OrganicAvenue.com

WWW.GlaserOrganicFarms.com

WWW.TheHealthyHaven.net

WWW.RawLife.com

WWW.EssentialLivingFoods.com

WWW.AlissaCohen.com

WWW.RawVolution.com

WWW.TheRawFoodWorld.com

WWW.GiveItToMeRaw.com

Personal Care Products

WWW.Aubrey-Organics.com

Raw Foods Educational Retreat Centers

WWW.HippocratesInst.com (Florida)

WWW.OptimumHealth.org (California and Texas)

WWW.TreeOfLife.nu (Arizona)

WWW.Wigmore.org (New Mexico)

WWW.CreativeHealthInstitute.us (Michigan)

WWW.AnnWigmore.org (Puerto Rico)

International

WWW.HappyCow.net

WWW.RawBC.org (Canada)

WWW.LivingFoods.co.uk (England)

WWW.EcoForest.org (Spain)

WWW.RawFoodMap.net (Scandinavia)

Sources Cited

Balch, Phyllis and James. *Prescription for Nutritional Healing* Third Edition. New York: Penguin Putnam, 2000.

Clement, Brian R. *Hippocrates Health Program,* West Palm Beach: Hippocrates Publications, 1992.

Cousens, Gabriel. *Spiritual Nutrition.* Berkeley: North Atlantic Books, 2005.

Furhman, Joel. *Disease Proof Your Child*, New York: St. Marks Press, 2005.

Heinerman, John. *Heinerman's New Encyclopedia of Fruits and Vegetables,* New Jersey: Prentice Hall, 1995.

Holford, Patrick. *Optimum Nutrition Bible,* Freedom: Crossing Press, 1999.

"24 Life-Extending Foods." *Hippocrates Newsletter.* (Vol. 24, Issue 2). West Palm Beach: Healthfulcommunications.com, 2005.

Leung, Albert. *Chinese Healing Foods and Herbs,* Glen Rock: AYSL ., 1984.

Howell, Edward. *Enzyme Nutrition.* New York: Avery, 1985.

Ludwig, Art. *Water Storage,* Santa Barbara: Oasis Design, 2005.

Morton, Julia F. *Fruits of Warm Climates.* Miami: Julia F. Morton, 1987.

Ody, Penelope. *The Complete Medicinal Herbal.* Dorling Kindersley, 1993.

Ross, Ivan A. *Medicinal Plants of the World.* New Jersey: Humana Press, 1999.

Index

Quotes

"When health is absent, wisdom cannot reveal itself, art cannot become manifest, strength cannot be exerted, wealth is useless and reason is powerless." Herophilies, 300 B.C.

"Remember, over 80 percent of all Americans die from cardiovascular disease, diabetes, and cancer, which are all diseases of nutritional ignorance." Joel Furhman, M.D.

"Nothing will benefit human health and increase the chances for survival of life on earth as much as the evolution to a vegetarian diet." Albert Einstein

"My refusing to eat meat occasioned an inconveniency, and I have been frequently chided for my singularity. But my light repast allows for greater progress, clearness of head and quicker comprehension." Benjamin Franklin

"Our bodies are our gardens, to which our wills are gardeners." William Shakespeare

"Water is the only drink for a wise man." Henry David Thoreau

"You are what you eat." American proverb

"People who don't have patience, become patients." Yogi Bhajan

"A closed mind is a wonderful thing to lose." Author unknown

"... vegetarianism should gradually eliminate the fierce and rugged elements from man's character, and fill the earth with gentle manners. It is both feasible and rational, and should appeal to and be practiced and advocated by all who seek the ideal life, and aim at producing a sweet-tempered, intellectual and artistic, yet vigorous, active and prolific race." Professor Gautier (quoted in *What To Eat In Health And Disease*, printed in 1923.)

"What people know depends on who owns the press." Bill Moyers

"Those who laugh, last!" Author Unknown

Who I am

I am letting go of who I was
So I can just be who I am.
Full speed ahead with this incarnation!
I am opening up to Life's inspiration.

A world full of promise, loving and giving
Comes alive inside me as I start forgiving-
Forgiving myself, for false imperfection
My sweet inner child has found Love's connection.

With new legs to lift me, I leap to the dance
Willing to risk, to dare for the chance-
The chance of a lifetime-
This lifetime to bring
Love where it isn't
And to write songs and sing!
To sing with the passion of love in my voice
That echoes the power of life's sacred choice-
To choose Love or choose fear,
The only choice that we're given
I choose Love!
I choose Love!
And thank God that I'm living.

-Rich Sommers